MARINE MEDICINE

ADVENTURE MEDICAL KITS

MARINE MEDICINE

A Comprehensive Guide

2nd Edition

- *Prepare for marine travel*
- *Identify hazardous marine life*
- *Learn over 50 improvised techniques*
- *Be safe—and confident!*

Eric A. Weiss, MD, FACEP
Michael E. Jacobs, MD, FAWM

THE MOUNTAINEERS BOOKS

To my wife, Genevieve,
our children and grandchildren,
and all those boaters I've had the opportunity to teach
or care for who have taught me so much in return. ❧
— M.J.

The Mountaineers Books
is the nonprofit publishing arm of The Mountaineers,
an organization founded in 1906 and dedicated to the exploration,
preservation, and enjoyment of outdoor and wilderness areas.

1001 SW Klickitat Way, Suite 201, Seattle, WA 98134

© 2012 Adventure Medical Kits

Second edition, 2012

Manufactured in the United States of America
Copy Editor: Heath Silberfeld, enoughsaid
Cover, Layout, and Book Design: Peggy Egerdahl
Illustrations: Gray Mouse Graphics, Moore Creative Designs, Rod Nickell,
    Danny Sun, Butch Collier, and Genevieve Jacobs
Cover photograph: *Man at the Helm of Yacht* © Mark Gerum/fstop/Corbis

Library of Congress Cataloging-in-Publication Data on file

ISBN (paperback):
    978-1-59485-660-0
ISBN (ebook):
    978-1-59485-661-7

SUSTAINABLE FORESTRY INITIATIVE
Label applies to the text stock

Certified Sourcing
www.sfiprogram.org
SFI-00341

CONTENTS

PREFACE

Dr. Eric Weiss's excellent book *Wilderness & Travel Medicine* is the solid foundation and structure for this book. This marine edition, *Marine Medicine: A Comprehensive Guide*, has been expanded to make it more relevant to the marine environment. The original content and concepts remain those of Dr. Weiss. This version contains references to sail- and powerboaters, white-water and flat-water paddlers, rowers, sea kayakers, surfers, and other water lovers who swim, scuba dive, snorkel, and generally enjoy all kinds of recreation on the water.

The illnesses and injuries suffered by these water sports enthusiasts are covered in detail. Material has been added to review medical evacuation at sea, marine communication, health and survival in a life raft, marine medical kits, submersion injuries, hazardous marine life, seafood poisoning, and many other medical emergencies and illnesses suffered by people in the aquatic setting. Sections on prevention of medical problems have also been added because preventing an illness or injury is, of course, the best medicine. The concept of prevention also applies to the early recognition and treatment of minor medical problems before they become major ones. The goal is to increase your self-reliance and medical skills so you are better able to do the right thing at the right time.

The information in these pages is intended to help you manage medical illnesses and emergencies in the marine environment when professional medical care or medical evacuation is not readily available. It is designed to help you evaluate a sick or injured person and handle a low-risk medical problem that you can safely and appropriately treat onboard, while avoiding an unnecessary and high-risk medical evacuation. The book is not a substitute for taking a comprehensive first-aid or wilderness medicine course, or for seeking prompt medical care in the event of a major illness or accident. Appendix C suggests organizations that provide training courses. Certification as a Wilderness Emergency Medical Technician (WEMT) or Wilderness First Responder (WFR) is most desirable in order to develop many of the skills and proficiency required for medical care in remote wilderness environments. Whenever someone becomes ill or injured, obtaining professional medical attention is a priority.

Use this book for guidance in difficult and remote situations, but do not attempt to perform any procedure that you are not comfortable with or trained to render, unless the person will die without that intervention. Legally, one is always liable for one's own actions, and one should never take any unnecessary risks or perform any medical procedure unless it is absolutely necessary.

Consult your physician about the medications you carry and inquire about potential complications or side effects, especially medications that can increase sensitivity to the sun (see Appendix B, page 306). Make sure you are not allergic to any drugs that you personally intend to use, and always inquire about possible allergies to any medication you may offer to someone else. Dispensing any medication to others is a serious responsibility and requires knowledge of the drugs and the illness being treated. Whenever possible, seek medical consultation before administering a prescription or nonprescription drug.

At the heart of wilderness and marine medicine is improvisation. In the wilderness (and remember, the sea is the greatest wilderness on Earth), one must utilize whatever supplies or materials are on hand, and depend heavily on common sense. Throughout this text you will find "Weiss Advice" features that describe improvised medical techniques. Most of these recommendations are supported by research published in medical journals. However, some are merely anecdotal, based on the author's experience and training.

Another feature is the "When to Worry" boxes, containing information that helps identify situations in which immediate evacuation is recommended. They provide only general guidelines, however, and ultimately the circumstance, combined with your own resources, training, and experience, should dictate your actions. When in doubt, it is always better to seek help rather than wait and see what happens.

May all your trips be safe, healthy, and filled with adventure!

Michael E. Jacobs, MD, FAWM

ACKNOWLEDGMENTS

I want to recognize my colleagues at the Wilderness Medical Society, who have been my mentors, educators, and supporters over the past three decades. During that time I have attended numerous educational meetings and have been given the opportunity to both help organize and participate in many conferences. I especially want to thank Drs. Paul Auerbach, Eric Johnson, Loren Greenway, Bill Forgey, Chris Van Tilburg, and the Society's stalwarts, Teri Howell and Jonna Barry. My special friend Chuck Hawley of West Marine has been my advisor and inspiration for the many courses we have taught together and the chapters and papers we have coauthored. I also recognize the special opportunity Dr. Peter Goth gave me when together we taught wilderness medicine for his new organization, Wilderness Medical Associates. Dr. Eric Weiss deserves special mention; he graciously agreed to coauthor this book on marine medicine using the foundation of his book, *Wilderness & Travel Medicine*. The Mountaineers Books have contributed their editorial and publishing expertise to make this second edition a high-quality and valuable book in any boater's library or medical kit. Adventure Medical Kits has continued to utilize this book in its marine medical kits and has supported the publishing of this second edition.

Michael E. Jacobs, MD, FAWM

HEALTH MAINTENANCE
The Fearsome Five: Food, Fluids, Fahrenheit, Fatigue, Fitness
"The Fearsome Five" identifies the issues that must be addressed in order to maintain the health and safety of all participants in marine activities, including the crew. A problem with any of the Fearsome Five will result in impaired physical and mental performance. To remain healthy in the wilderness environment, one requires sufficient fuel in the form of nutritional *food* to maintain energy and normal body functions; adequate amounts of clean drinking *fluids* to prevent dehydration; protection from the elements (sun, wind, water, spray, cold, and heat) to maintain normal body temperature *(Fahrenheit)*; sufficient time to nap, sleep, or rest in order to overcome *fatigue*; and training to prevent injury and illness *(fitness)*. This all may sound simple and obvious, but in austere settings and environmental extremes, these five areas become the focal points not just for personal performance but for survival. This guide addresses many of these issues. Concentrate on the Fearsome Five during your excursions on the water, and you should remain well and return in good, if not better, health.

TRAUMATIC INJURIES: WHERE TO BEGIN
The ABCs of Marine First Aid: The Primary Survey
Wilderness medicine encompasses nine immediate priorities, regardless of the injury or illness. The acronym "ABC" is a helpful mantra for recalling the nine priorities in the order that they are performed. The nine priorities define an expanded "primary survey" and encompass a rapid evaluation of the scene and the person in which life-threatening conditions, such as a blocked airway, severe bleeding, and cardiac arrest, are recognized and immediate treatment is rendered.

The ABCs	
A1	**ASSESS** the scene
A2	**AIRWAY** (ensure an open airway)
A3	**ALERT** others
B1	**BARRIERS** (protect rescuer with gloves, mask)
B2	**BEGIN** rescue breathing/CPR
B3	**BLEEDING** (stop bleeding)
C1	**COMPLETE** a secondary survey
C2	**CERVICAL** spine protection (prevent unnecessary movement of the head and neck and protect the spine)
C3	**COVER** and protect the person (from the environment)

A1: Assess the Scene

Always ensure the safety of the uninjured crew/trip members first. Before rendering medical care, assess the scene for further hazards, such as equipment failure, changing weather, sea or river conditions, or changes in the boat's seaworthiness. Do not allow your sense of urgency to ignore addressing conditions that might endanger yourself or the crew.

A2: Airway

Make sure the person is breathing and does not have an obstructed airway. Speak loudly to the person as you approach. A response indicates that the person is breathing and has a pulse. For infants and children, gently tap them on their hands and feet and call their name. If

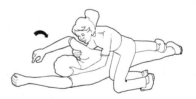

Fig. 1 *Single rescuer logrolling a victim faceup without twisting the spine*

unresponsive, immediately determine if the person is breathing. If facedown, logroll the person onto the back so that the head, shoulders, and torso move as a single unit without twisting (**Fig. 1**). Place your ear and cheek close to the person's mouth and nose to detect air movement, while looking for movement of the chest and abdomen (**Fig. 2**). In cold weather, look for a vapor cloud and feel for warm air movement.

If the person is not breathing, or has noisy (obstructed) breathing, clean the mouth out with your fingers and open the airway. If you do *not* suspect trauma, the airway can be opened by placing the palm of one hand on the forehead and tilting the head back while the fingers of the other hand lift the chin (**Fig. 3**). The most common reason for an airway obstruction in an unconscious person is relaxation of the muscles of the tongue and throat, which allows the tongue to fall back and block the airway.

If the person is unconscious after trauma (e.g., due to a head or spine injury from the boom), use the jaw-thrust technique, which minimizes movement of the neck and spine, to open the airway. The jaw thrust is performed by kneeling down with your knees on either side of the person's head, placing your hands on either side of the person's jawbone, and pushing the base of the jaw up and forward (**Fig. 4**). If you do not detect breathing after opening the airway or observe only occasional gasps (agonal respiration), presume that the person is in cardiac/respiratory arrest, immediately alert others, and initiate CPR (see "Cardiopulmonary Resuscitation [CPR]," page 24).

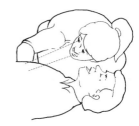

Fig. 2 *Checking for breathing*

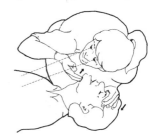

Fig. 3 *Opening the airway of an unconscious victim when trauma is not suspected*

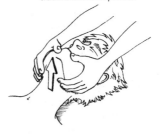

Fig. 4 *Using the jaw-thrust technique to open the airway after trauma*

☀ Weiss Advice

Opening the Airway with Two Safety Pins

Keeping the airway open with the jaw-thrust technique occupies both your hands. If you are by yourself, an airway can be kept open by pinning the front of the person's tongue to the lower lip with two safety pins (**Fig. 5a**). An alternative to pinning the lower lip is to pass a string or shoelace through the pin in the tongue, keeping the tongue forward by tying it to the person's shirt button or jacket zipper (**Fig. 5b**).

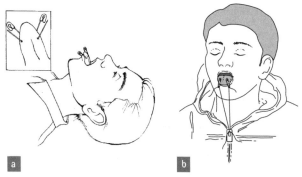

Fig. 5   *Tongue traction: An alternative to piercing the lower lip is to pass a string through the safety pins and exert traction on the tongue by securing the end of the string to the victim's shirt button or jacket zipper.*

A3: Alert Others

Before becoming more involved with the resuscitation, take a few moments to call or signal for help. Assign a crew member to activate the red "distress" button on a VHF radio enabled for Digital Selective Calling (DSC), the Coast Guard's new marine radio network, or transmit a Mayday call on channel 16 (the distress channel) of an older-model

VHF radio. "Mayday" is the top-priority distress signal if someone is in imminent danger and requires immediate assistance. Urgent, non-life-threatening emergencies are prefaced with the signal "Pan-Pan" (pronounced pahn-pahn). Seeking medical evacuation for a sick or injured crew member falls into this category. In other settings, activating an emergency position-indicating radio beacon (EPIRB) might be appropriate (see "Calling for Help by Radio," page 43 and "Calling for Help by Cell Phone, Satellite Phone, and Emergency Beacons," page 45). If a radio or satellite or cell phone is not available, use the maritime distress signals (see Appendix H, page 322).

B1: Barriers

Any time you deal with blood or bodily fluids, it is vitally important to protect yourself from the germs in blood, urine, and saliva, which transmit diseases such as hepatitis and HIV. Protect your hands with virus-proof gloves and use a barrier device when performing mouth-to-mouth rescue breathing. Even nitrile gloves can leak, so make sure you wash your hands or wipe them with an antimicrobial towelette after removing the gloves.

WARNING: Latex allergies can produce skin rashes, severe anaphylactic reactions, and death. If you suspect that you or the victim might have an allergy to latex, use powder-free nitrile gloves.

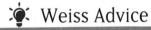

☀ Weiss Advice

Improvised Barrier

Any gloves are better than using your bare hands. Dishwashing gloves make an effective barrier to blood. An improvised glove can also be made by placing your hand inside a sandwich or garbage bag and securing it to your wrist with tape or string.

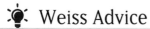

Weiss Advice

Improvised Barrier for Mouth-to-Mouth Breathing

A glove can be modified and used as a barrier shield for performing rescue breathing (**Fig. 6**). Simply cut the middle finger of the glove at its halfway point and insert the glove into the person's mouth. Stretch the glove across the person's mouth and blow into the glove as you would to inflate a balloon. The slit creates a one-way valve, preventing backflow of the person's saliva.

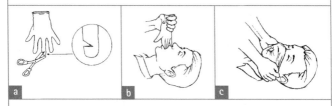

Fig. 6 *Improvised glove barrier*

B2: Begin Rescue Breathing/CPR

Recognition of cardiac arrest is not always a straightforward matter for untrained medics. If after the airway is open a person is unresponsive with no breathing or abnormal breathing (e.g., only gasping), immediately begin CPR. Trained medics should take no more than 10 seconds (30 seconds if the person is severely hypothermic) to check for a pulse. Place your index and middle fingers on the person's throat over the Adam's apple, and then slide your fingers down the side of the person's neck to the space between the Adam's apple and neck muscle to feel the

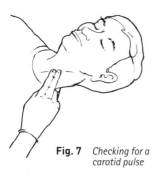

Fig. 7 *Checking for a carotid pulse*

carotid pulse (**Fig. 7**). If you do not detect a pulse, initiate CPR (see "Cardiopulmonary Resuscitation (CPR)," page 24).

If the person does not breathe independently after establishing an airway but has a pulse, begin mouth-to-mouth rescue breathing (see "Rescue Breathing," page 27). Immediately after being hit by lightning or immediately after inhaling water during a submersion incident, a person may require only rescue breathing (and not the chest compressions of CPR), because the heart may not have stopped beating and will continue to beat if breathing is quickly restored.

B3: Bleeding

Check the person for signs of profuse bleeding. Then, with a gloved or protected hand, remove clothing and check the entire person for signs of bleeding. Arterial bleeding may be recognized because it often spurts as the heart beats. Trying to judge by color whether the source of blood is a vein or artery is essentially impossible. To stop bleeding, use your gloved hand to apply pressure with a dressing directly to the wound (**Fig. 8**).

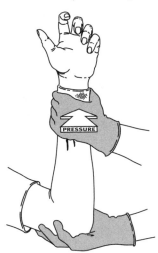

If bleeding from an extremity cannot be stopped by direct pressure and the person is in danger of bleeding to death, apply a tourniquet (**Fig. 9**). A tourniquet is any band applied around an arm or leg tightly enough that all blood flow beyond the band is stopped. If the tourniquet is left on for more than 4 hours, the arm or leg beyond the tourniquet may die and require amputation. Damage to the arm or leg is rare if the tourniquet is left on less than 2 hours.

Fig. 8 *To stop bleeding, use your gloved hand to apply pressure directly to the wound.*

In the face of massive extremity hemorrhage, it is better to accept the small risk of damage to the limb than to have a person bleed to death (see "Controlling Bleeding," page 120).

How to Apply a Tourniquet

1. Tourniquet material should be at least 5 cm (2 inches) wide and flat, to prevent crushing tissue. Use a firm bandage, belt, or sail tie that will not stretch. Never use wire, thin line, or any material that will cut the skin.
2. Wrap the bandage snugly around the extremity several times as close above the wound as possible (between the wound and the heart), and tie an overhand knot.
3. Place a stick or similar object on the knot, and tie another overhand knot over the stick.
4. Twist the stick until the bandage becomes tight enough to stop the bleeding. Tie or tape the stick in place to prevent the tourniquet from unwinding.
5. Note the time the tourniquet was applied.
6. If you are more than an hour from medical care, loosen the tourniquet very slowly at the end of 1 hour, while maintaining direct pressure on the wound. If bleeding is still heavy, retighten the tourniquet. If bleeding is then manageable with direct pressure alone, leave the tourniquet in place, but do not tighten it again unless severe bleeding starts.

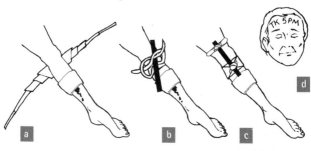

Fig. 9 *Applying a tourniquet*

C1: Complete a Secondary Survey

Once you have made sure that no life-threatening issues require attention, perform a head-to-toe examination of the person, looking for additional injuries. Gently push on every part of the person, assessing for tenderness, swelling, instability, or deformity. Obtain vital signs, mental status, and organize your evaluation (see "The Secondary Survey," page 38).

C2: Cervical Spine Protection

The spinal cord is vital for life; it runs down from the brain through the vertebrae in the neck to the lower back. Spinal cord damage can cause permanent paralysis or death. It is necessary to immobilize the spine to prevent further injury after an accident that could have broken the person's neck, such as a fall, head injury, or shallow-water diving accident, and if any of the following are present:

- The person is unconscious, and therefore you cannot perform a reliable exam.
- The person complains of neck or back pain.
- There is tenderness in the back of the neck or upper back when pressing the bumps and depressions along the spine.
- There is numbness, tingling, or altered sensation in the extremities (the person is unable to feel light touch, a painful pinch, or a pinprick).
- The person is unable to move or has weakness in an arm, hand, finger, or leg that is not due to direct injury to that part.
- The person has an altered level of consciousness, or is under the influence of drugs or alcohol, and the examination is unreliable.
- A very painful injury—such as a thigh (femur) or pelvis fracture, dislocated shoulder, or broken rib—may distract the person from noticing neck pain.

If a cervical spine injury is suspected, the medic should immobilize the person's head and neck, and prevent any movement of the torso. Avoid moving someone with a suspected spine injury if the person is in a safe location. Transfer the person in a full body litter. (See "Treatment of Specific Fractures: Neck and Spine Fractures," page 91.)

C3: Cover and Protect the Person
In a cold environment, place insulating garments or blankets underneath and on top of the person for protection from hypothermia. Use a sail bag or foul-weather gear for added protection. Remove any wet clothing, dry the skin, and replace with dry clothing. In a hot environment, loosen the person's clothing and create shade. If the person is in a dangerous or exposed area, initiate removal to a safer location while maintaining, if indicated, spine immobilization.

LIFE-THREATENING EMERGENCIES I:
CPR, RESCUE BREATHING, AND CHOKING

Cardiopulmonary Resuscitation (CPR)
New guidelines by the American Heart Association recommend that the three steps of cardiopulmonary resuscitation (CPR) be rearranged. The new first step is doing chest compressions instead of mouth-to-mouth breathing. This does not apply to submersion incidents, where rescue breathing is still an essential part of CPR. The new guidelines apply to adults, children, and infants, but they exclude newborns.

When to Start and Stop CPR
Do not be afraid to start CPR, fearing that you might be criticized for not continuing it indefinitely. It is impossible to know exactly how long a person found unconscious and without a pulse has actually been in cardiac arrest. In the wilderness and at sea, if CPR (performed for any reason) is not successful in resuscitating the person after 30 minutes, and the person is not severely hypothermic, you may discontinue the effort.

- Do not begin CPR where you face threats, such as dangerous sea conditions requiring the crew to manage the boat.
- Do not begin CPR if it diverts attention from other injured persons who have a greater chance of survival.
- CPR probably should not be attempted following cardiac arrest caused by severe traumatic injury.
- CPR should be continued beyond 30 minutes following hypothermic cardiac arrest *only* if the individual can be subsequently evacuated to a medical center for rewarming and continued critical care.

Only four conditions appear to justify trying CPR at sea. Success with CPR following the first three situations is limited, and care for other individuals with life-threatening conditions should take precedence.

- Persons struck by lightning who have not been breathing for less than 10 minutes (These individuals may need only rescue breathing.)
- Witnessed drowning
- Unwitnessed drowning in cold water when the rescued person's pulse and respiration were initially present at the time of recovery and then ceased
- Witnessed collapse from cardiac arrest

CPR: Infants Younger Than 1 Year

1. Try to wake the infant by rubbing the soles or tapping on the shoulder or chest. Do not shake a baby.
2. If the infant is not breathing, put two fingers on the breastbone directly between the baby's nipples. Push straight down about 4 cm (1.5 inches) or about one-third of the thickness of the baby's chest, and then let the chest rise all the way back up. Do this 30 times, about twice per second.
3. After pushing on the chest 30 times, cover the baby's entire mouth and nose with your mouth, and gently blow until you see the chest rise. Let the air escape—the chest will go back down— and give one more breath.
4. Continue the compression-to-breathing ratio of 30 compressions for every two breaths.
5. Don't stop until the baby wakes up or starts breathing independently.

CPR: Adults and Children Older Than 1 Year

1. If you find an unresponsive person (i.e., no movement or response to stimulation) or witness an individual who suddenly collapses, attempt to wake the person by tapping on the shoulder and shouting. If the person also has absent or only occasional gasping breathing, assume that the person is in cardiac arrest. If you are trained in how to detect a pulse, take no more than 10 seconds to check for a pulse (30 seconds if the person is severely

hypothermic) and, if you do not definitely feel a pulse within that time period, start chest compressions.

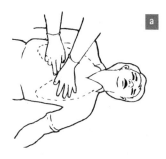

2. Place the person faceup on a firm surface. Place the heel of your hand in the middle of the person's chest and put your other hand on top of the first with your fingers interlaced (**Fig. 10**).

3. Compress the chest at least 5 cm (2 inches). Allow the chest to completely recoil before the next compression. Your shoulders should line up directly over the person's breastbone, with elbows straight.

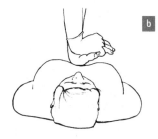

4. Keeping your arms stiff and using a smooth motion, compress the breastbone at a rate of at least 100 pushes per minute. That's about the same rhythm as the beat of the Bee Gees' song "Stayin' Alive" (**Fig. 11**). Do not remove your hands from the person's chest between compressions. You may feel

Fig. 10

Place the heel of one hand in the middle of the chest. Place the other hand on top with fingers interlaced. Your shoulders should line up directly over the victim's breastbone.

pops and snaps when you first begin chest compressions—don't stop! You're not going to make the person worse.

5. After 30 compressions, open the person's airway using the head-tilt, chin-lift method (**Fig. 12**). Pinch the person's nose, and make a seal over the person's mouth with yours. Use a CPR mask if available or improvise one from materials at hand (**Fig. 6**, page 20).

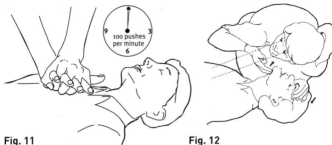

Fig. 11
Keeps arms stiff and compress the breastbone at a rate of at least 100 pushes per minute.

Fig. 12
Opening the airway of an unconscious victim when trauma is not suspected

Give the person a breath big enough to make the chest rise. Let the chest fall, then repeat the rescue breath once more. If the chest doesn't rise on the first breath, reposition the head and try again. If you don't feel comfortable with this step, just continue to do chest compressions at a rate of at least 100 per minute without rescue breathing (hands-only CPR).

6. Use a compression-to-breathing ratio of 30 chest compressions for every two breaths.

7. If two medics are working together, switch off doing compressions and breathing every 2 minutes to prevent fatigue. Check every 5 minutes for the return of a pulse or spontaneous breathing.

Rescue Breathing

Rescue Breathing: Children Older Than 1 Year

1. Cover the child's mouth with your mouth. Pinch the child's nose closed with the thumb and forefinger of your hand that is on the forehead for the head tilt. Use your other hand to lift the chin (**Fig. 13**).

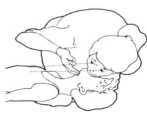

Fig. 13 *Rescue breathing, child*

2. Breathe two slow breaths (1 to 1.5 seconds in length) into the child's mouth, with a 2-second pause between breaths. Breathe enough air in to make the child's chest rise.
3. If the child does not start to breathe independently, check for a pulse. If a pulse is present, continue rescue breathing with 20 breaths per minute. If no pulse is present, start chest compressions.

Rescue Breathing: Adults

1. Check for breathing. If not lying faceup, gently roll the person over, moving the entire body as a unit while supporting the spine.
2. If no breathing is detected, open the airway with the head-tilt maneuver. Place the palm of one hand on the forehead and tilt the head back while the fingers of the other hand grasp and lift the chin (**Fig. 12**, page 27).
   Note: If a neck injury is suspected, use the jaw-thrust technique to open the airway (**Fig. 4**, page 17). Sweep two fingers through the person's mouth to remove any foreign material or broken teeth.
3. If the person does not start to breathe independently, pinch the nostrils closed and place your mouth over the mouth (**Fig. 14**).
   A CPR face shield or modified glove (see Weiss Advice: Improvised Barrier for Mouth-to-Mouth Breathing, page 20) can be used during mouth-to-mouth rescue breathing to prevent physical contact with the person's mouth.
4. Blow air into the person until you see the chest rise. Remove your mouth to allow the person to exhale. Give two initial breaths: one before and one after allowing the person to exhale.
5. Repeat this procedure, giving a vigorous breath every 5 seconds until the person starts to breathe

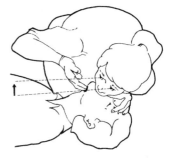

Fig. 14 *Rescue breathing, adult*

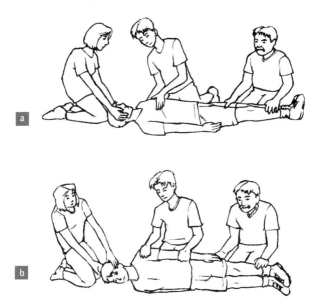

Fig. 15 *Logrolling a victim onto their side for vomiting or to place a board or insulation under the victim*

spontaneously, help arrives, or you are too exhausted to continue.

6. If air does not move in and out of the person's mouth easily or if the chest does not rise, first try tilting the head farther back, or if a cervical spine injury is suspected, repeat the jaw-thrust technique, pushing the person's jaw farther out. If breathing still does not occur, the airway may be obstructed by a foreign body (see "Choking/Obstructed Airway," page 30).

7. During mouth-to-mouth rescue breathing, the person's stomach will often fill with air, eventually resulting in vomiting. If vomiting occurs, logroll the person in a manner that maintains spine alignment, and clear the airway (**Fig. 15**).

Choking/Obstructed Airway

Choking is a life-threatening emergency that occurs when something blocks the person's airway and prevents breathing. Choking should be suspected when an individual suddenly becomes agitated and clutches the throat, especially while eating. The person may be unable to speak and then become cyanotic (turn blue).

Choking: Adults and Children (Heimlich Maneuver)

1. Stand behind the person and wrap your arms around the person's waist. Make a fist with one of your hands and place it just above the person's navel and below the rib cage, with the thumb side against the abdomen.
2. Grasp your fist with your other hand and pull it forcefully toward you, into the person's abdomen and slightly upward with a quick thrust. If unsuccessful, repeat the procedure (**Fig. 16**).

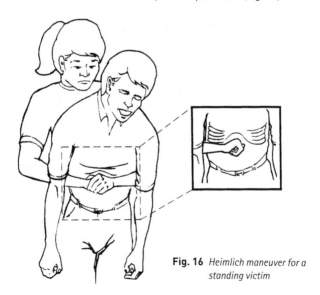

Fig. 16 *Heimlich maneuver for a standing victim*

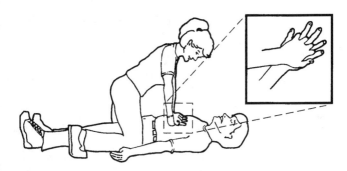

Fig. 17 *Heimlich maneuver for an unconscious adult*

If the adult or child becomes unconscious:
1. Lay the person faceup and attempt rescue breathing (see "Rescue Breathing," page 27).
2. If you cannot get air into the person and/or the chest does not rise with rescue breathing, perform the Heimlich maneuver while kneeling and straddling the person's thighs. Use the heel of your hand instead of your fist (**Fig. 17**).
3. If still unsuccessful, look for foreign material in the person's mouth and, if found, remove it. Continue to perform the Heimlich maneuver and periodically attempt rescue breathing. If multiple attempts at clearing the airway and breathing air into the person are unsuccessful, a surgical airway (cricothyroidotomy) is indicated.

Surgical Airway (Cricothyroidotomy)
A cricothyroidotomy is a technique that allows rapid entrance to the air passage in a person who is unable to breathe from a blocked airway. It is a very challenging and potentially complication-prone procedure, but one that may be lifesaving. It should be attempted only after trying the Heimlich and other noninvasive techniques to relieve the obstruction in the airway have been exhausted, and the victim is on the verge of dying from lack of air.

In the wilderness, a cricothyroidotomy is done by cutting a hole in the thin cricothyroid membrane of the windpipe (trachea) and then placing a hollow object into the trachea to let air enter the lungs. The cricothyroid membrane lies just below the Adam's apple in the center of the neck and feels like a small depression between the Adam's apple and the firm ring below it (the cricoid cartilage).

How to Perform a Cricothyroidotomy

1. With the person lying faceup, clean the neck around the Adam's apple with an antiseptic if one is readily available. Put on protective gloves (see "How to Put On Surgical Gloves," page 68).
2. Find the Adam's apple with your finger (this is the most prominent firm structure in the center of the neck). Slowly run your finger downward toward the chest (keeping your finger in the midline of the neck) until you feel a small indentation between the bottom of the Adam's apple and the top of the cricoid cartilage (the next firm and prominent structure that you feel as you move down

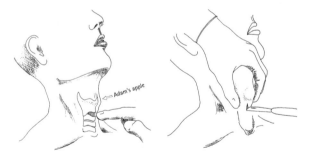

Fig. 18 *Location of the cricothyroid membrane just below the Adam's apple in the midline of the neck*

Fig. 19 *Making a vertical 2.5-cm (1-inch) incision through the skin over the cricothyroid membrane*

Continued

the neck). The indentation between the Adam's apple and the cricoid cartilage in the windpipe, called the cricothyroid membrane, is the spot that you want to puncture (**Fig. 18**).

3. Make a vertical 2.5-cm (1-inch) incision with a knife through the skin over the membrane (go a little bit above and below the membrane) while using the fingers of your other hand to pry apart the skin edges. Anticipate bleeding from the wound. After the skin is cut apart, puncture the membrane by stabbing it with your knife or other pointy object, e.g., a marlin-spike (**Fig. 19**).

4. Stabilizing the windpipe between the fingers of one hand, insert a hollow object—such as the barrel of a syringe (see right), ballpoint pen casing, or stiff straw (**Figs. 20–21**)—through the membrane with your other hand. Secure the object in place with tape.

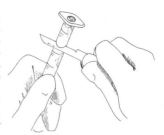

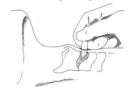

Fig. 20 *Cutting the barrel of a 1-cc or 3-cc syringe at a 45 degree angle*

Fig. 21 *Inserting a hollow tube through the cricothyroid membrane*

5. Breathe air into the person through the object, as if you were blowing through a straw, and then remove your mouth to allow exhaled air to exit. Repeat this step at the same frequency as if you were performing mouth-to-mouth rescue breathing.

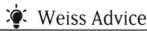

Weiss Advice

Using a Syringe as a Breathing Tube

Remove the plunger from the barrel of a 3-cc or 1-cc syringe. Using a sharp knife or saw, cut the barrel at a 45-degree angle at its midpoint to create an improvised airway for inserting through the cricothyroid membrane (**Figs. 20** and **21**, page 33).

LIFE-THREATENING EMERGENCIES II: HEART ATTACK, STROKE, SHOCK, AND ANAPHYLACTIC SHOCK

Heart Attack

A heart attack occurs when the blood supply to the heart muscle is reduced or completely blocked due to an obstruction in one of the arteries supplying blood to the heart. If blood flow is not restored within 1 to 6 hours, part of the heart muscle will die.

Signs and Symptoms

The primary symptom of a heart attack is chest pain. The pain is usually a pressure, crushing, tightness, or squeezing sensation located in the center of the chest, and it may radiate up into the neck and jaw or shoulders, or down the arms. Sometimes the person experiences a burning sensation in the lower chest near the stomach or a feeling of indigestion. Cold sweats, nausea, vomiting, anxiety, shortness of breath, and weakness are often present.

Treatment

1. Administer 1 aspirin tablet (325 mg) to the person immediately. Have the person either chew or crush and then swallow the tablet. Continue to give $^1/_2$ tablet daily. Aspirin may help to partially open the blocked artery.
2. Let a person who has nitroglycerin tablets take them as prescribed.
3. If your advanced medical kit contains clopidogrel (Plavix) 75 mg, administer 4–8 tablets at once, then 1 daily. This drug helps to stop complete blockage of the artery.

4. If your advanced kit contains metoprolol (Toprol) 25 mg, then give 1 tablet every 6 hours. This drug helps to reduce the workload on the heart.
5. If available, administer oxygen and pain medication to the person.
6. Keep the person at rest in a comfortable position.
7. Arrange immediate evacuation to a medical facility.
8. There is no reason to carry a defibrillator when cruising or paddling in remote areas. This equipment is indeed lifesaving only in the context where medical help and advanced cardiac life support are promptly available.

When Risk of Heart Disease Is Higher

If you are traveling or cruising with people with a higher risk of heart disease, consider stocking aspirin 325 mg, nitroglycerin tablets, clopidogrel (Plavix) 75 mg, metoprolol (Toprol) 25 mg, oxygen, and pain medication.

Stroke

A stroke is a life-threatening event in which an artery to the brain bursts or becomes clogged by a blood clot, cutting off the supply of oxygen to a part of the brain. A stroke can affect the senses, speech, behavior, thought patterns, and memory. It may also result in paralysis, coma, and death.

Signs and Symptoms

Any or all of the following may occur during a stroke:

- Sudden weakness or numbness of the face, arm, and leg, usually on one side of the body (One side of the person's mouth may appear to droop.)
- Loss of speech or trouble talking or understanding speech
- Loss of vision in only one eye
- Sudden dizziness or loss of coordination
- Sudden onset of a severe headache

Treatment

The person should be evacuated to a medical facility. Continually reassess the person's airway and level of consciousness, as the condition can dramatically worsen during transport.

Shock

Shock is a life-threatening condition in which blood flow to the tissues of the body is inadequate and cells are deprived of oxygen. Any serious injury or illness can produce shock. Examples are severe bleeding (hemorrhagic shock), which may be internal bleeding (e.g., a ruptured spleen) or external bleeding (e.g., a thigh or pelvis fracture); dehydration; heart failure (cardiogenic shock); severe allergic reactions (anaphylactic shock); severe infections (septic shock); or spinal cord injuries with paralysis (spinal shock).

Signs and Symptoms

The skin is pale, cool, or clammy. The pulse is weak and rapid, or even undetectable (in shock produced by a spinal cord injury, the pulse will remain normal or slow). Breathing may be shallow, rapid, or irregular. Mental status may be altered (the person may be confused, restless, or combative). Blood pressure is always below normal.

Treatment

It is important to recognize shock, stabilize the person, and arrange evacuation to a medical facility.

1. Keep the person lying down, covered and warm, and well-insulated from the underlying surface.
2. Stop obvious bleeding.
3. Loosen restrictive clothing.
4. Splint all broken bones. If the femur is fractured, apply and maintain traction (see "Weiss Advice: Traction Splint," page 105). If a pelvic fracture is suspected, apply a pelvic wrap (see "Pelvic Fractures," page 103).
5. Elevate the legs so that gravity can help improve the blood supply to the heart and brain, only if external bleeding has been controlled. If the person has internal bleeding, avoid unnecessary movement and keep the person lying flat. For cardiogenic shock,

the person may be more comfortable with the head and chest raised slightly to allow easier breathing.

6. If anaphylaxis is suspected, treat immediately with epinephrine (see "Anaphylactic Shock," below).

7. If dehydration is suspected and the person is awake, begin oral or other routes for hydration (see "Weiss Advice: Rehydration Solutions," page 172).

Anaphylactic Shock

The most severe form of allergic reaction is anaphylactic shock, which can be life-threatening within minutes after contact with the substance to which the individual is allergic.

Signs and Symptoms

The person may develop hives (red, raised skin welts), wheezing, chest tightness, shortness of breath, and a drop in blood pressure leading to dizziness, light-headedness, and fainting. The soft tissues of the throat, larynx, or trachea may swell, making it difficult or impossible for the person to swallow, speak clearly, or breathe.

Treatment

The treatment for anaphylactic shock is epinephrine (adrenaline), and it needs to be given immediately. This drug is an essential part of the medical kit.

People allergic to bee stings or with other serious allergies should carry injectable epinephrine with them at all times. Epinephrine requires a prescription and is available in an injectable cartridge called the EpiPen or EpiPen Jr Auto-Injector. It allows for self-administration of the medicine quickly without dealing with a separate vial, needle, and syringe. The device contains 2 mL of epinephrine 1:1000 USP in a disposable push-button, spring-activated cartridge with a concealed needle. EpiPen will deliver a single dose of 0.3 mg epinephrine intramuscularly. For children who weigh less than 30 kg (66 pounds), the EpiPen Jr, which contains half the dose of the adult injection (0.15 mg epinephrine), is used. Instructions for use accompany the kits. After administering epinephrine, give the person oral diphenhydramine (Benadryl) 25 to 50 mg, a popular antihistamine that may lessen the allergic reaction.

After treatment, transport the person to a medical facility immediately; an anaphylactic reaction can recur once the epinephrine wears off, in which case the dose can be repeated if the reaction is severe.

THE SECONDARY SURVEY

Once you have completed the primary survey and made sure that there are no life-threatening problems, begin the secondary survey. Training is recommended in order to perform this evaluation with a high level of skill and confidence. This is a focused history and physical exam, together with a measurement of the vital signs (if not already completed). This information will help you formulate an assessment of the problem and a plan for treatment.

Definition of Signs and Symptoms

Diagnosis of an injury or illness relies on the ability to examine the person thoroughly and identify the important medical clues referred to as signs and symptoms.

Signs are what you observe when you examine a person with your eyes, ears, nose, and hands. For example, you might see bluish discoloration of the skin, hear labored or noisy breathing, smell pus in a wound infection, or feel swelling under the skin.

Symptoms are what the person tells you he or she is experiencing, such as pain, nausea, dizziness, or headache.

Physical Exam

In cases of trauma, perform a complete, hands-on, head-to-toe examination of the person, looking for evidence of injury. Look at, feel, and gently press on every part of the person, checking for bleeding, open wounds, discoloration, swelling, lumps, pain, tenderness (pain caused by touch), instability, deformity, or muscle spasm. Note if there is a lack of circulation, numbness, or an inability to move the affected part. The examined area must be exposed, and it may be necessary to cut away clothing to avoid moving the injured area. Compare what appears abnormal to the opposite, unaffected part of the body. Talk with the person during the entire exam, tell the person what you are doing, and ask about pain, discomfort, and any abnormal sensations (e.g., numbness) as you examine the person.

When there is a specific illness or limited injury (e.g., abdominal pain, finger mashed in a winch), perform a more focused examination of the affected area by looking for signs and symptoms. Examination of the entire body is not always necessary.

Vital Signs

Measurement of vital signs may help to identify problems, and will certainly help determine if a person is stable, deteriorating, or improving in response to treatment. This information may guide you and those assisting by radio or phone about the necessity for urgent medical evacuation. Vital signs should be recorded, along with the time they are obtained; they should be obtained as frequently as the problem requires or the condition of the person changes. Vital signs consist of the following:

- *Pulse:* The heart rate per minute. Normal adult rate is 60–85 beats per minute. Use the radial pulse on the thumb side of the inner wrist. Count for a minute (or 30 seconds and multiply by 2).
- *Respiration:* Normal adult rate is 12–20 respirations (breaths) per minute. Note if respiration appears labored or easy and natural.
- *Blood Pressure* (BP): Normal adult BP is 110/60 to 140/90, but it varies widely among healthy people. Blood pressure, reliably measured with a blood pressure cuff and stethoscope, is a skill that requires training. Small, portable devices to measure blood pressure are also available for laypersons.
- *Temperature:* Normal body temperature is 36.6–37.2°C (98–99°F). It is most useful to know temperature when evaluating the degree of hypothermia and hyperthermia (along with the signs and symptoms). Use a thermometer designed for low temperature readings when evaluating hypothermia, and take the temperature rectally (this temperature may not be completely reliable).
- *Skin:* Color, temperature, and moisture of the skin are also vital signs. Note if the skin is warm or cool to touch, wet or dry, and if it is pale. Blue areas (cyanosis) in the lips or nail beds indicate poor circulation.
- *Level of Consciousness and Mental Status:* Note if the person is awake, unconscious (unresponsive), or somewhere in-between

(responds to his or her name or to a pinch). If the response to questions is reasonably coherent and appropriate, then mental status is normal.

History

Very often, people will tell you what is ailing them and will lead you to the correct diagnosis. Give them time to describe their condition (symptoms) and listen carefully and patiently without interrupting. Try to obtain a past medical history, including a list of current medications and known allergies.

Organizing Your Thoughts and Information

Organized medical information gathered through the history, physical examination, and vital signs is the ideal foundation for communicating with medical consultants. Only relevant information should be included. Without experience and training, observation may be imprecise and a diagnosis impossible, so just do the best you can. The better you communicate, the more likely an appropriate plan of action can be formulated. The goal is to avoid a hazardous medical evacuation for a medical problem that can be treated on the scene, and to prevent minor problems from becoming more serious. The ultimate objective is to do the right thing at the right time.

An example of a concise radio message to the medical control officer at a Coast Guard station, or to a physician you call on a radio or satellite phone, might be as follows:

History: "At 12:30 PM, a 32-year-old man fell overboard without a life jacket after he slipped on deck. We recovered him within 10 minutes. He quickly came to the water surface, but he feels he inhaled some water. He is complaining of difficulty breathing and feels short of breath."

Physical: "Vital signs: pulse 120; respiration 22; blood pressure not obtained; temperature not obtained: skin color normal. He is awake. Breathing appears difficult, not easy, and he is coughing white sputum. I put my ear to his chest, and the breathing is noisy."

Assessment: "Not sure what is going on. Is there water in the lungs?"

RESCUE AND EVACUATION OF THE SICK AND INJURED

After consultation and assessment of the person's medical problem, a plan to either evacuate the person or continue medical care must be formulated. The decision is based on the nature of the illness or injury, availability of rescue personnel and craft, proximity to a medical facility, and the medical expertise of the crew. When at sea, transferring personnel from a boat to a rescue ship or helicopter entails risk for everyone. It may well be the most dangerous aspect of the ordeal. A leader should be designated to oversee the entire process and delegate responsibilities for the care of the person and coordination of the medical evacuation. A team approach is essential.

Offshore, merchant ships may be the only option for a medical evacuation. In ship-to-ship rescue, collision between the smaller vessel while alongside the larger ship is the greatest risk. Be prepared to damage your vessel in this situation. The typical scenario is a large merchant ship with very limited maneuverability approaching a smaller vessel. Unless the ship is designed for rescue work, the captain and crew experienced, and the seas relatively calm, it is much safer for the boats and crew to use a smaller craft (lifeboat, dinghy, or even a life raft) to transfer the person between the two boats. These smaller craft can be hoisted up to the deck of the rescue ship with a hoist or cargo crane.

Helicopter Rescue and Safety

Helicopter emergency evacuation and rescue efforts have now become commonplace within 482 km (300 miles) of the coastal United States and may be available in national parks, national scenic river corridors, and other wilderness areas. Consider helicopter rescue when medical treatment is urgently needed. Radio or phone consultation with the rescue coordination center will help determine the feasibility, appropriateness, and logistics of evacuating a person.

Safety Rules

On Land:
1. Maintain radio contact with the pilot to advise about local weather conditions and landing zone.
2. Stand outside the landing zone, with your back to the prevailing wind, and face the approach path.
3. Remove loose debris and supplies from the landing zone.
4. Keep in full view of the pilot and crew. Do not approach the helicopter until signaled by the crew.
5. Stay clear of the tail rotor; approach from the downhill side of any slope, always toward the side of the helicopter, and never from directly in front.

At Sea:
1. Listen for pilot's radio briefing on VHF channel 16.
2. Secure all loose gear on deck.
3. All personnel on deck should wear life jackets.
4. Place wind 45 degrees off the port bow.
5. Avoid shining a flashlight directly at the helicopter.
6. Never fire aerial flares in the vicinity of the helicopter.

Note: Most of the time a rescue swimmer from the helicopter will come aboard and assist in all of the following maneuvers.

7. Tend the orange steadying line dropped from the helicopter to guide the litter onto the deck; it is safe to hold.
8. Discharge static electricity by allowing the metal litter or hoist cable to initially contact the water or boat.
9. Unhook the hoist cable from the litter before moving it.
10. Never attach the hoist cable or any line from the helicopter to the boat.
11. *When evacuating someone on a litter*, put a life jacket on the person, then wrap the evacuee in a tarp or blanket and secure the person in the litter with the straps provided. *When evacuating someone in a helicopter's rescue basket or horse collar sling*, put the person in a life jacket.

Calling for Help by Radio

Within 40 km (25 miles) of the coastal United States, the marine VHF-FM radio is the most popular and reliable tool for ship-to-ship communication and for contacting the nearest Coast Guard operations center. The VHF signal range is limited to line of sight and therefore depends on the height of both the transmitting and receiving antennas. The range may extend up to 482 km (300 miles) when communicating with an aircraft. A transmission range of 24 to 32 km (15 to 20 miles) can be expected between boats with masthead-mounted antennas; powerboats have half the range. A portable handheld VHF unit can transmit up to 8 km (5 miles) over water to another VHF radio or to a coastal relay station.

The new Rescue 21 system relies on VHF radios and the new Digital Selective Calling (DSC) standard as the preferred hailing system for transmitting Mayday calls and for establishing voice radio communication on the marine VHF band. VHF radios with this DSC feature can automatically send out a distress message with the push of a red "distress" button to staffed Coast Guard shore stations as well as Coast Guard and other vessels in radio range. This technology enables the Coast Guard to obtain multiple lines of bearing to a Mayday call and determine with precision the location of the vessel in distress. No special license or training is required to use the radio other than reading the manufacturer's instruction booklet, perhaps taking a 20-minute online tutorial, and registering the radio for a Maritime Mobile Service Identity (MMSI) number. The radio can be linked to an onboard GPS unit to automatically broadcast the location of the boat together with the emergency call.

Understanding and Using a VHF Radio

- Place a call for assistance as early as possible during an emergency, and assign a crew member to monitor radio contact.
- Turn power on and adjust the volume. Turn the squelch control knob clockwise until the static noise disappears. Keep the radio antenna of a portable radio vertical and a few inches away from your mouth; speak across the mouth area, not directly at it.
- Transmit a distress call on VHF channel 16. All sets have a designated button that immediately selects this channel; switch to another frequency if later instructed to do so.

- Set transmit power to high. Use low power to contact nearby boats.
- Depress the call button on the microphone to transmit, and keep it depressed throughout your message; release the button to hear a response. You cannot transmit (talk) and receive (listen) at the same time.
- Speak slowly and distinctly, with normal voice and volume. Keep your communication simple and concise.
- Know or estimate the boat's location before commencing transmission. Refer to any recognizable landmarks onshore. Ask the radio contact to repeat your location back to you to avoid error.
- Use the appropriate alerting signal. "Mayday" is the top-priority distress signal if the crew is in imminent danger and requires immediate assistance. Urgent but not life-threatening emergencies are prefaced with the signal "Pan-Pan" (pronounced pahn-pahn). Seeking medical evacuation for a sick or injured crew member falls into this category.
- When using the handheld portable radio, stand up and get as high as possible. This will extend the line of sight an additional 1.5 to 3 km (1 or 2 miles).
- If there is no response to the message, wait 5 minutes with the radio on, and then repeat the call.

The DSC VHF radio has some additional operation features that you should become familiar with if this type of radio is onboard your boat.

How to Make a Distress Call or Request a Medical Evacuation
Communicate who you are, where you are, and what's wrong.
- "Mayday, Mayday, Mayday" or "Pan-Pan, Pan-Pan, Pan-Pan"
- "This is vessel ___ ." Repeat the name three times.
- "We are located ___ ." Give the most accurate position.
- "We need assistance for ___ ." Specify the nature of the medical problem.
- "The boat is ___ ." Give a full description of the craft (type, color, size), including any distinguishing characteristics.

- "There are ___ people onboard." State the total number of individuals.
- "This is ___ (repeat the boat's name) standing by on channel ___."
- End the message by saying "Over."
- Repeat this call and listen for a response between transmissions.

Calling for Help by Cell Phone, Satellite Phone, and Emergency Beacons

When you're in trouble, a cell phone may not help. The average effective range for a cellular phone offshore is 16 km (10 miles); use is restricted to high-traffic areas where there are both cellular antennas and relay stations. A cell phone may function in harbors and near shore, but it is useless on the high seas. Area geography can also block a cell phone signal, making the phone unusable.

Cell phones have additional disadvantages. The Coast Guard's radio direction finders (RDFs) cannot determine the caller's location from a cell phone call. Calls to 911 from maritime locations may be misdirected to police or fire departments, which may delay water rescue responses. The privacy of cell phone communication, in contrast to the open party-line communication of VHF radio is the real problem: it excludes potential emergency assistance from boats in the vicinity who may overhear your call while monitoring VHF channel 16. Cell phones also do not enable the caller to be contacted by rescue boats or aircraft that use VHF radios.

Iridium or Inmarsat satellite phones with worldwide coverage are ideal for their portability, cost, and ease of operation. Like any other portable phone, a crew member can immediately use it. (See Appendix J, page 324 for the locations of the U.S. Coast Guard Rescue Coordination Centers and their phone numbers.) A phone can be purchased or rented with a waterproof case, which makes it ideal for inclusion in an "abandon ship" bag.

A satellite phone is also an excellent choice for emergency voice communications from remote areas (e.g., wilderness rivers, backcountry lakes) where cell phones and portable VHF, UHF, and HF radios cannot connect to their network signal or are beyond useful range.

A personal locator beacon (PLB) with integrated GPS is another option. It transmits a distress signal and precise location on 406 MHz to orbiting satellites, which then relay the information to appropriate rescue coordination centers. As a last resort, a PLB can be activated in situations where a person or group is in grave and imminent danger, or where urgent medical attention is required. It is an electronic Mayday call, without voice communication. PLBs must be registered with NOAA to identify the owner and obtain a unique identification number, which is encoded in the signal.

HEAD INJURIES

Head trauma and brain injury can result from direct impact or from the shearing forces produced by rapid deceleration. When your head hits a hard object, such as a boulder, or is struck by a flying boom, the impact can fracture the skull, bruise the brain, or cause severe bleeding inside the brain from damaged blood vessels. Shearing forces from sudden deceleration of the brain against the inside of the skull can also tear blood vessels on the surface of the brain, leading to an expanding blood clot and pressure on the brain (intracranial pressure).

Rising intracranial pressure is bad for several reasons. The increased pressure makes it difficult for the heart to pump enough blood to the head. This is a catastrophe for the brain, which depends on a constant supply of blood to bring it oxygen and other nutrients. If the pressure within the skull rises high enough, it can force parts of the brain downward through the base of the skull (herniation), causing damage to the brain structures and, ultimately, death. Compression of one of the nerves as the brain swells produces dilatation of one or both pupils, an important sign of a severe head injury. Head injuries can be subdivided into different categories based on their severity.

Severe Head Injury: Prolonged Loss of Consciousness

Loss of consciousness for more than 5 to 10 minutes or an altered level of consciousness (person is only responsive to verbal arousal or painful stimuli) following a head injury is a sign of significant brain injury. Assess the person's airway and perform rescue breathing if necessary. Because of the potential for accompanying neck and spine injuries with severe head trauma, the person's spine should be immobilized. As soon as possible, evacuate the person to a medical facility and maintain spine immobilization. Be prepared to logroll a vomiting person onto the side. Continually monitor the airway for signs of obstruction (listen for noisy or labored breathing) and a decreasing respiratory rate. Keep the person warm and dry and be prepared for progressive neurological deterioration.

Mild Head Injury: Brief Loss of Consciousness

Short-term unconsciousness, in which the person wakes after 1 or 2 minutes and gradually regains normal mental status and physical abilities, is evidence of a concussion. A concussion does not usually produce permanent damage, although confusion or amnesia about the event and repetitive questioning by the person are common. The person may feel stunned and disoriented initially, but brain function is normal. A concussion represents a diffuse traumatic injury to the brain, and potential injury to the spine, face, and skull should still be evaluated.

To be safe, if on land or in harbor, evacuate the person to a medical facility for evaluation. Boaters should head for harbor, or at a minimum, while at sea, keep the person under close observation for at least 24 hours, and do not allow the person to perform potentially hazardous activities. Begin radio communication to alert nearby boats and potential medics of the situation and the possible need to evacuate the person if the condition worsens. Normal sleep should be interrupted every 3 to 4 hours to check that the person's condition has not deteriorated and that he or she can be easily aroused. If the person becomes increasingly lethargic, confused, or combative; is just not acting as you would expect; or develops any of the other signs of head injury (see "When to Worry: Head Injury Checklist," page 48), evacuation should take place as soon as possible.

Getting plenty of rest and sleep helps the brain to heal. Keep the person warm, hydrated, and fed. Avoid situations that could produce a subsequent head injury, and consult with a physician before returning to contact sports. A repeat concussion that occurs before the brain has fully healed can be very dangerous and may slow recovery or increase the chance for long-term problems. Most persons with a concussion recover quickly and fully. During recovery, many people have a range of symptoms that may appear right away, or they may not be noticed for hours or even days after the injury.

Head Injury with No Loss of Consciousness

If an individual suffers a head injury but never loses consciousness, remains awake and alert, has no amnesia, and has normal neurological function, the injury is rarely serious. Although a mild headache, bleeding from a scalp wound, or a large bump on the head may be evident, evacuation isn't necessary unless the person develops any of the problems listed in the checklist below.

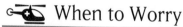 # When to Worry

Head Injury Checklist

Seek immediate medical attention if any of the following symptoms occur after a blow to the head:

- A headache progressively worsens.
- Consciousness gradually deteriorates from alertness to drowsiness or disorientation. Ask the person his name, the location, the date, and what happened. Getting all four correct means the person is "oriented x 4." Getting three correct but not knowing what happened indicates a possible concussion.
- Persistent or projectile (shoots out under pressure) vomiting occurs.
- One pupil becomes significantly larger than the other.
- Bleeding from an ear or nose occurs without direct injury to those areas, or a clear watery fluid drains from the nose.
- Bruising is visible behind the ears or around the eyes, when there is no direct injury to those areas.
- Seizures occur.

Prevention of Head Injuries

Prevention for Sailors

The mainsail boom is the number one cause of head injuries on a sailboat, and the majority of boom-related head injuries are fatal. The spinnaker boom at the bow may swing wildly if unattended during sailing maneuvers. Accidental jibes result when the wind from astern (behind the boat) causes the sail and boom to suddenly swing across the cockpit and deck. A crew member unaware of the jibe can be struck in the head or chest. Simple sailing maneuvers, such as changing course, can threaten any crew member unaware of a swinging boom approaching at head level. Rigging failures may cause the mast to fall to the deck and cause head and other injuries.

Carelessly stored or unsecured objects in the cabin or in unlatched lockers are another hazard. They become flying missiles as the boat rolls or capsizes, and head injury often results.

- Be attentive and be aware of wind direction. Watch the boom while on deck and during all sailing maneuvers. If you must take your eyes off the boom, keep low and out of its path while it swings.
- When sailing off (away from) the wind, use a boom preventer (a line secured from the end of the boom to the bow) to avoid accidental jibes.
- The crew should practice sailing maneuvers and sail changes in heavy weather and limited visibility to avoid head injury from trips, falls, and collisions with each other on deck.
- Regularly inspect rigging, lines, and blocks (pulleys) for wear.
- Secure supplies in drawers and lockers with strong, properly fitted latches to prevent accidental opening and the contents becoming flying missiles.

Prevention for Paddlers

Head trauma occurs in river rafting, kayaking, and canoeing when capsized boaters strike rocks in fast-moving water.

- White-water boaters should wear undamaged, correctly fitted helmets. Wear helmets while scrambling over slippery or unstable boulders on a riverbank.
- Paddlers should be skilled in self-rescue techniques, including escape from an overturned craft and white-water swimming strategies. Use legs as shock absorbers if unable to swim aggressively to shore. In rapids, lie on your back with your feet on the surface pointed downstream. Remember that the current flows around rocks, so go with the flow until it is safe to eddy out.

Prevention for Surfers

Head injuries; scalp lacerations; concussions; nasal, tooth, and jaw fractures; and ruptured tympanic membranes are frequent injuries among surfers. Surfboard fins or a blunt part of the board striking a surfer on the head is usually the cause.

■ Use small, light boards with surfboard leashes, which prevent loose boards from striking other surfers. Rubberized nose guards and tail guards applied to the nose and tail of the board reduce injury. Foam boards with soft fins are safer for beginners.

Head and spinal cord injuries are common while bodysurfing, especially among those surfing hollow shore breaks. These injuries happen as a surfer pitches forward and lands headfirst on a hard or sandy bottom.

■ Wear a snug surfing helmet, especially when surfing over shallow reefs or in crowded conditions.

■ If you feel yourself going over the falls, lead with a shoulder, not your head.

Prevention for Swimmers and Divers

■ Use caution when diving into a pool, pond, or river. Only dive into water you know to be deep enough and free of underwater hazards.

■ Ascend from a scuba dive looking up toward the surface with an arm extended overhead to avoid hitting a floating object or the dive boat.

Skull Fractures

Fracture of the skull is not life-threatening unless associated with underlying brain injury, spine injury, or severe bleeding.

Signs and Symptoms

Signs of a skull fracture include a sensation that the skull is uneven when touching the scalp, blood or clear fluid draining from the ears or nose (without direct trauma to those areas), and black-and-blue discoloration around the eyes (raccoon eyes) or behind the ears (Battle's sign).

Treatment

Evacuate the person to a medical facility as soon as possible for evaluation.

Scalp Wounds

Scalp lacerations are common after head injuries, and they tend to bleed a lot because of their rich blood supply. Fortunately, applying direct pressure to the wound with a gloved hand can usually stop bleeding. It might be necessary to hold pressure for up to 30 minutes (see "Using Staples to Close a Wound," page 130).

☀ Weiss Advice

Hair-Tying a Scalp Wound Closed

If you're faced with a bleeding scalp wound and the injured person has a healthy head of hair, you can tie the wound closed using the person's own hair (**Fig. 22**). Take a piece of dental floss, sail thread, or regular sewing thread and lay it on top of, and parallel to, the wound. Twirl a few strands of hair on each side of the wound, then cross them over the wound in opposite directions, forcing the wound edges closed. Have an assistant tie the strands of hair together with the dental floss or thread while you hold the wound closed with the strands of hair. A square knot works best. You can also use a drop of superglue to hold the strands of hair together. Repeat this technique as many times as necessary along the length of the wound until the cut is closed.

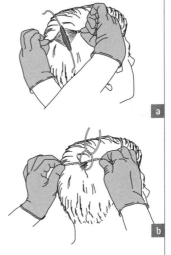

Fig. 22 *Hair-tying a scalp wound closed*

EYE AND NOSE INJURIES
Eye Trauma
Signs and Symptoms

If the eye is hit, a visible layer of blood may settle behind the cornea (the transparent front part of the eye that covers the colored iris and black pupil) during the next 6 to 8 hours. Treat by patching the eye closed with a gauze pad and tape. Seek medical care as soon as possible, keeping the head elevated and in an upright position.

If the eyeball is perforated (ruptured), the person will experience loss of vision ranging from blurred sight to total blindness. Other signs and symptoms include pain, an unchanging wide dilated pupil, and blood in the eye.

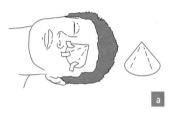

Trauma to the eye can also cause the retina to become detached from the back of the eye. Symptoms include persistent light flashes and floating spots in the field of vision. Vision loss is physically painless. A detached retina requires surgical repair. Seek immediate medical care.

Do not rinse the eye or try to remove any object stuck into the eyeball. Cover the eye with a paper cone, cup, or other protective object and secure this protective covering in place with a bandage (**Fig. 23**). Be careful not to put pressure on the eye. If possible, patch both eyes or have the person keep both eyes closed to avoid movement of the injured eye. Evacuate the person to a medical facility as soon as possible. If evacuation is delayed more than 6 hours, start antibiotic

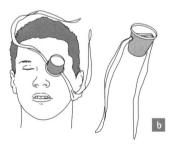

Fig. 23 *Two different techniques for improvising and securing a protective cover for a perforated or ruptured eye*

therapy with amoxicillin clavulanate (Augmentin), cephalexin (Keflex), or azithromycin (Zithromax, Zmax).

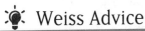

Weiss Advice

Relieving Eye Pain

Drops of tea squeezed from a cool, nonherbal tea bag may help to soothe the eye and relieve pain.

Scratched Eye (Corneal Abrasion)

The cornea is a thin, clear, protective shield at the front of the eye. It covers the colored part of the eye and the pupil. A corneal abrasion is a scratch on the cornea. It can be caused by something blowing into the eye, or by something rubbing across the cornea.

Prevention
- Wear protective eye goggles while working with tools that cause bits of wood, paint chips, or other material to fly into the air. Eye injuries are common while doing maintenance work on boats (scraping, sanding, painting, etc.)
- Watch for low-hanging tree branches when approaching a riverbank from the water. Helmets, visors, and hats decrease visibility in such circumstances.
- Use care when replacing contact lenses that may shift while swimming.
- Wear sunglasses when boating and walking on beaches and riverbanks.

Signs and Symptoms
- The person feels as if sand is in the eye.
- The eye appears bloodshot, and there is often tearing and slight blurring of vision.
- Intense pain, made worse by blinking the eyes, may occur, and there is sensitivity to light.
- Close inspection of the cornea may show a slight irregularity on its surface.

Treatment

1. Check the eyes carefully for foreign material, making sure to examine under the upper lid (see "Superficial Foreign Bodies," page 55).
2. Cool compresses may help relieve some of the irritation.
3. Instill antibiotic eyedrops such as ofloxacin (Floxin) ophthalmic drops every 2 to 3 hours while awake for 2 to 3 days. Antibiotic ointment can also be used. Apply a ribbon of erythromycin 0.5% ophthalmic ointment four to six times daily along the margin of the lower lid.
4. Administer oral pain medication (ibuprofen [Advil, Motrin]) and rest the eyes as much as possible. Most of the time, the injury heals by itself in 1 to 2 days.
5. Contact lens use increases the risk of eye infection. Remove contact lenses immediately and reinsert them after the abrasion heals (48 to 72 hours) and the antibiotic course is completed. Seek consultation if symptoms worsen within 3 to 4 hours of lens removal.
6. Eye patching is no longer routinely recommended for corneal abrasions. The patch itself may be the main cause of pain, retard the healing process, and increase the chance of infection. Wear sunglasses to protect the eye from wind and sun.
7. Any worsening of symptoms should prompt a thorough reinspection for foreign bodies and infection, followed by a consultation.

⌖ When to Worry

Scratched Eye

Seek medical care immediately if the person has a scratched eye and any of the following signs or symptoms:

- The injury does not improve and heal in 2 to 3 days.
- There is increasing redness, pain, or swelling.
- Greenish fluid begins to drain from the eye.
- The person's vision worsens.

☀ Weiss Advice

Improvised Sunglasses

If you forget or lose your sunglasses, you can cut slits in a piece of card-board, such as one side of a cracker or cereal box, or a piece of duct tape folded back over onto itself. These should be just wide enough to see through (**Fig. 24**). Tape or tie this around your head to minimize the amount of ultraviolet light hitting your eyes.

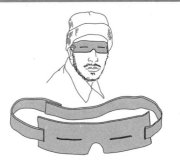

Fig. 24 *Improvised sunglasses*

Subconjunctival Hemorrhage

Small blood clots on the white part of the eye sometimes occur after physical exertion or coughing. Parts of the white of the eye become bright red. It looks like a serious condition, but it is not. The eye is not painful, and vision is normal. The hemorrhage will resolve on its own in a few weeks.

Superficial Foreign Bodies

The best method for removing a speck of dirt from the eye is to let the eye tear. Irrigating the eye with clean water or eyewash under slight pressure using a syringe or a soft water bottle is an option if the particle remains in place. Another technique is to have the person immerse the face in a basin of clean water, or grossly clean river or lake water, and open the eyes while blinking; this should wash out the irritating material. After irrigation, gently pull the lids away from the eye while the person looks up, down, left, and right. Use a flashlight and magnifying glass if necessary. Remove any residual material with a moistened cotton-tipped applicator, cloth, or gauze, then pull down the lower lid, and apply erythromycin ophthalmic ointment.

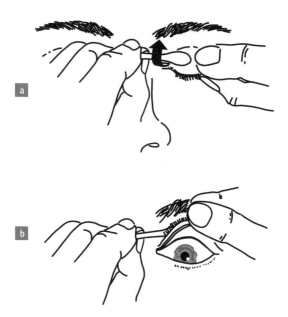

Fig. 25 *Everting the eyelid with a cotton-tipped applicator to locate a foreign body*

Sometimes the foreign body will lodge underneath the upper eyelid. To examine under the upper lid, have the person look downward as you grasp the eyelashes with your thumb and finger. Place the cotton end of a cotton-tipped applicator in the middle of the upper lid. Using the applicator as a fulcrum, pull the lid forward and upward, causing it to fold back over the applicator (inside out) while exposing the undersurface of the lid (**Fig. 25**). The foreign object can then be removed with the corner of a moistened cloth or a cotton swab. After objects are removed from the eye, persons often report feeling as if something is still in the eye. Small scratches on the surface of the cornea usually cause this. Treat this the same as for a scratched eye (see "Scratched Eye," page 53).

☀ Weiss Advice

Eye Irrigation

Pour disinfected water into a clean sandwich or garbage bag and puncture the bottom of the bag with a safety pin. Squeeze the top of the bag firmly to create an irrigation stream, which can then be directed into the eye.

Burns of the Eye

The eye can be injured from accidental splashes while handling battery acid or specific cleaning agents (e.g., bilge cleaner, paint solvents). The eye becomes painful, tears, and may turn red or white. Regardless of the offending agent, treat by thoroughly flushing the eye for a minimum of 30 minutes with clean fresh water. Clear (not murky) seawater is also acceptable. Make sure the fluid gets behind the upper and lower eyelids. Apply a topical anesthetic if available, followed by antibiotic ointment, and eye patch. A minor burn is self-limiting; more severe burns require consultation.

Nosebleeds

The great majority of nosebleeds originate from the front of the nose and respond well to simple treatment. This area is susceptible to bleeding after facial trauma, and to injury (drying out) in hot, dry environments. Have the person recline, keeping the head elevated, and gently blow the nose to remove residual clots and blood. This blood is dark and comes out with small clots. Dripping bright red blood signifies active bleeding.

Pinching the soft part of the nostrils together between thumb and index finger and holding firmly for at least 15 to 20 minutes usually can control nosebleeds. If blood continues to drain down the back of the throat despite pinching the nostrils tightly, it indicates a posterior (back of the nose) bleed. This is a serious problem, as the person can lose a significant amount of blood and it can interfere with breathing. If the bleeding does not stop on its own after a few minutes, you may need to pack both the front and back of the nose (see "Weiss Advice," pages 58 and 59). If the bleeding stops when you pinch the nostrils but resumes when you let go after 20 minutes of firm pressure, you may need to pack only the front of the nose.

☀ Weiss Advice

Packing the Front of the Nose

If bleeding cannot be controlled by pinching the nostrils together for a full 20 minutes, nasal packing should be considered (**Fig. 26**).

1. If available, first insert into the nose a piece of cotton or gauze soaked with a blood vessel constrictor such as oxymetazoline nasal spray (Afrin), leave it in place for 5 minutes, and then remove it.

2. Cut a large gauze pad or soft cotton cloth into a thin continuous strip and coat this with petroleum jelly or antibiotic ointment (**Fig. 26a**).

3. Gently pack it into the nostril, using tweezers or a thin twig so that both ends of the packing material remain outside of the nasal cavity. Start the packing with the middle of the strip. This will keep the packing from going down the back of the throat. To completely pack the nasal cavity of an adult, you will need about 1 m (3 feet) of packing (**Fig. 26b**).

4. Secure the ends of the pack to the face with tape (**Fig. 26c**).

5. Leave the pack in for 24 to 48 hours, and then gently remove it. If bleeding starts again, repack the nostril.

6. Packing the nose will block sinus drainage and predispose the person to a sinus infection. Antibiotics such as amoxicillin clavulanate (Augmentin), cephalexin (Keflex), or azithromycin (Zithromax, Zithromycin) should be taken until the packing is removed.

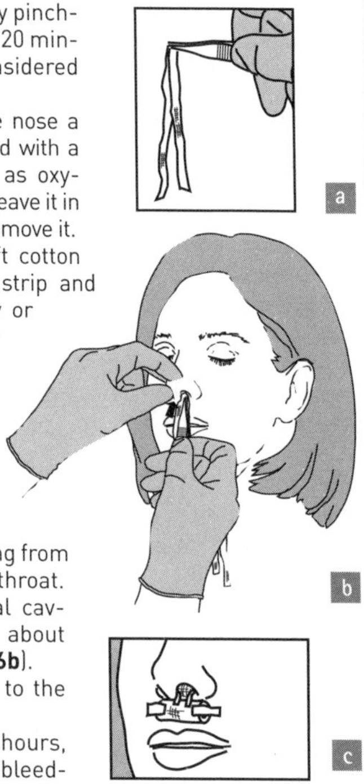

Fig. 26 *Packing the front of the nose*

🔆 Weiss Advice

Packing the Back of the Nose

Bleeding from the back of the nose can be difficult to control and requires a posterior pack. A 5-mm (14–16 French) Foley catheter (something you may want to add to your first-aid kit) can be used to pack the back of the nose.

1. First, lubricate the catheter with either petroleum jelly or antibiotic ointment, then insert it through the nasal cavity to the back of the throat. (If the victim's mouth is open, you should be able to see the tip of the catheter in the throat behind the tongue. [**Fig.27a**]) Inflate the balloon of the catheter with 10 to 15 mL of air from a syringe.
2. Then gently draw the catheter out of the nose until resistance is met (**Fig. 27b**).
3. Secure the catheter firmly to the victim's forehead with several strips of tape.
4. Pack the front of the nose (as described on the previous page).

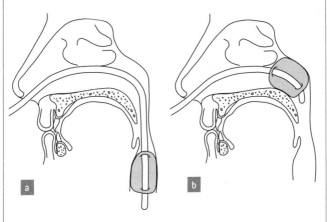

Fig. 27 *Packing the back of the nose*

DENTAL INJURIES AND EMERGENCIES
Toothache

The common toothache is caused by inflammation of the dental pulp and is often associated with a cavity.

Signs and Symptoms
The pain may be severe and intermittent, and is made worse by hot or cold foods or liquids.

Treatment
1. If the offending cavity can be localized, a piece of cotton soaked with a topical anti-inflammatory agent, such as oil of cloves (eugenol) can first be applied.
2. Place a temporary filling material, such as Cavit or zinc oxide and oil of cloves cement, into the cavity or lost filling site to protect the nerve.

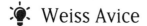 **Weiss Avice**

Replacing a Lost Filling

Melt some candle wax and allow it to cool until it is just soft and pliable. Place the wax into the cavity or lost filling site and smooth it out with your finger. Have the person bite down to seat the wax in place, then remove any excess wax.

Dental Infections and Abscesses
Signs and Symptoms
Dental pain associated with swelling in the gumline at the base of the tooth might indicate a tooth infection or abscess. Tapping the offending tooth causes pain, but the tooth should not be sensitive to hot or cold. Dental infections occasionally spread beyond the tooth to the floor of the mouth, face, and neck. If this occurs, the person may have difficulty opening the mouth, swallowing or breathing, and fever and swelling of the face may develop.

Treatment

Dental infections can lead to serious illness and often require intravenous antibiotics, as well as extraction of the tooth or root canal therapy. Swelling of the face indicates a serious spreading infection. If a dentist cannot be reached, start oral antibiotics (penicillin 500 mg, four times a day, or amoxicillin clavulanate [Augmentin] 875 mg, twice daily) and warm-water mouth rinses.

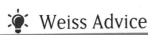 Weiss Advice

Relieving Dental Pain and Bleeding with a Tea Bag

Pain and bleeding from the mouth can often be relieved by placing a moistened nonherbal tea bag onto the bleeding site or into the socket that is bleeding. Leave it in place for 5 to 10 minutes.

Displaced Tooth

If a tooth is knocked out, it may be salvageable if replaced within 30 to 60 minutes. A child's primary tooth should not be placed back in the socket.

Treatment

1. Handle the tooth only by the crown and not by the root.
2. Clean the debris off the tooth by rinsing gently (do not scrub!) with saline, milk, or disinfected water, and gently place the tooth back into the socket.
3. If the tooth cannot be replaced immediately, store it in a container containing saline, milk, or saliva, in that order of preference.

Loose Tooth

A tooth that becomes loosened, but not displaced, due to trauma should be repositioned with gentle, steady pressure. A soft diet should be maintained to avoid any further trauma until the tooth heals. See a dentist as soon as possible for definitive treatment.

CHEST INJURIES: RIB FRACTURES

A forceful blow to the chest or a fall on a boat's deck may break one or more ribs. Broken ribs are very painful but usually require only pain medication and rest. Sometimes, the complications may be life-threatening and difficult to diagnose.

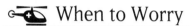 # When to Worry

Chest Injuries

One end of a broken rib can sometimes be displaced inward and puncture the lung, producing a pneumothorax (see "Collapsed Lung [Pneumothorax]," page 65). Rib fractures can also bruise the lung or predispose the person to pneumonia. If a lower rib is fractured, it may injure the spleen or liver and cause severe bleeding. Multiple rib fractures can produce a flail chest (see "Flail Chest," page 64). Evacuation to a medical facility as soon as possible is indicated if the person has more than one rib fracture, or if the person develops shortness of breath, difficulty breathing, persistent cough, fever, abdominal pain, or dizziness or light-headedness upon standing.

Prevention

Sailors often suffer chest injury when the boat's motion becomes erratic or the decks become slippery. Falling onto a winch, vent, stanchion, cleat, windlass, or any of the many protruding objects on deck and belowdecks can easily break a rib and/or damage the lungs. Taking the following preventive measures can reduce serious trauma:

- Crouch and lower your center of gravity when walking aboard a rolling, pitching boat or any small unstable craft (e.g., rowboat, small open motorboat).
- Wear nonskid, well-fitted footwear.
- Use a safety harness aboard a sailboat as a "third hand" when working on deck in rough weather.
- Place grab rails in strategic locations on deck and belowdecks. Apply nonskid adhesive pads to ladders and other frequently wet and slippery surfaces.
- Illuminate the deck when walking on deck at night.

- In rough weather, wear a float coat or comfortable life vest to provide padding and protection to the rib cage.
- Use lee cloths or boards to secure sleeping sailors in their bunks while underway. Pillows and blankets can provide additional padding.
- Remove or lower the oarlocks in rowboats before moving in or out of them.
- Walk up and down companionway steps while facing the ladder and holding onto the railings.
- Rib fractures are the most common fracture in windsurfers. The majority of rib injuries result from contact with the boom, which occurs from high-speed falls or catapults. Catapulting occurs in gusty winds when sailors are unable to disengage the harness rapidly and are launched into the air, often landing on the boom or mast. Know how to disengage a harness to prevent chest injury and sail within your level of expertise, especially when using the harness.

Signs and Symptoms
- Chest pain made worse by taking a deep breath
- Chest pain made worse by certain movements
- Extreme tenderness at the fracture site
- A crackling or grating sensation or sound can occasionally be detected upon touching the broken rib
- Rib fractures usually occur along the side of the chest. Pushing on the breastbone (sternum) while the person lies faceup will produce pain at the fracture site rather than at the breastbone.

Treatment
Oral pain medication ibuprofen [Advil, Motrin]; or acetaminophen with hydrocodone [Vicodin]) will help reduce pain and make breathing easier. After the pain is relieved, encourage hourly deep breathing and coughing to keep the lung expanded. It takes about 2 weeks for pain to subside and 4 to 6 weeks for the rib to heal. Taping the chest over the fractured rib or lying on the injured side while the area is being splinted can provide added pain relief. A simple, uncomplicated rib fracture does not require medical evacuation.

Flail Chest

When three or more consecutive ribs on the same side of the chest are broken in two places, a free-floating segment called a flail chest can result. The underlying lung is usually bruised.

Signs and Symptoms

The flail segment will move opposite to the rest of the chest during breathing and make it hard for the person to get enough air. The movement of broken ribs causes great pain, which further reduces the person's ability to breathe.

Treatment

1. Evacuate the person to a medical facility as soon as possible. A flail chest can be tolerated only for the first 24 to 48 hours, after which the person will usually need to be put on a ventilator to assist with breathing.
2. The flail segment must be immobilized at once. Gently place a bulky pad of dressings, rolled-up extra clothing, or a small pillow over the site, or splint the arm against the injury with something soft and lightweight to stabilize the flail segment and relieve some of the pain. Use large strips of tape to hold the splint in place. Do not tape entirely around the chest, as this will further restrict breathing. The main function of this splint is to make it less painful to breathe, not to stop movement of the chest or restrict breathing in any manner.
3. Administer pain medication.
4. Transport a person who is unable to walk by either lying them face up or on the injured side. Allow the person to assume the most comfortable position for breathing.
5. If the person is severely short of breath and cannot get enough air, you may need to assist the breathing with mouth-to-mouth rescue breathing. Time your breaths with the person's, and breathe gently to provide added air with each inspiration.

Collapsed Lung (Pneumothorax)

A collapsed lung occurs when air enters the chest cavity and compresses or collapses the lung. This can occur when a broken rib punctures the lung, an outside object such as a knife penetrates the chest, or even spontaneously, when a weak point develops in the lung and permits air to leak into the chest cavity. A pneumothorax can develop if a scuba diver ascends to the surface too rapidly (see "Barotrauma: Injuries of Ascent," page 251).

Signs and Symptoms
- Sharp chest pain, which may become worse with breathing
- Shortness of breath or difficulty breathing
- Reduced or absent breath sounds (place your ear on the chest wall of the person) together with diminished chest movement on the injured side

Treatment

Evacuate the person and monitor closely for the development of a tension pneumothorax.

Tension Pneumothorax

A pneumothorax can progress to a life-threatening condition called a tension pneumothorax if air continues to leak into the chest cavity. With each breath, air enters the space surrounding the lung, but it cannot escape with exhalation. Pressure soon builds up, compressing the lung and heart, which can eventually lead to death.

Signs and Symptoms
- Labored breathing, air hunger, and agitation
- Cyanosis (bluish skin discoloration)
- Signs of shock (weak and rapid pulse; rapid breathing; agitation; pale and moist skin; and confusion)
- Visibly bulging veins on each side of neck (jugular veins)
- Diminished or absent breath sounds on the injured side (place your ear on the chest wall of the person)

- Bubbles of air felt or heard under the skin (crackling) on touching the chest wall, areas above collarbone, or neck
- Visible or palpable deviation of the trachea to one side of the neck
- Heart sounds shifted from normal location on left side of the chest

Treatment

If the situation is desperate and the person is literally dying before your eyes, you can do only one thing to possibly save the life: you must relieve the pressure from inside the chest (pleural decompression) and allow the lung to re-expand. This procedure takes courage and improvisation in the wilderness or onboard a boat at sea. Pleural decompression should not be undertaken casually and should be attempted only if the person appears to be dying. Possible complications include infection; profound bleeding from puncture of the heart, lung, or a major blood vessel; or even laceration of the liver or spleen—all of which may cause death.

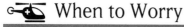 # When to Worry

Hemorrhage and Shock
A person with an open chest wound below the nipple line may also have an injury to an abdominal organ such as the spleen or liver. Internal bleeding and hemorrhagic shock can result.

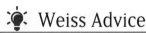 Weiss Advice

How to Perform Pleural Decompression

Note: This should not be undertaken casually.
1. Swab the skin between the collarbone and the nipple on the side of the procedure with 10% povidone-iodine (Betadine) or another antiseptic.
2. If sterile gloves are available, put them on after washing your hands (see "How to Put On Surgical Gloves," page 68).
3. If local anesthesia is available, inject it into the skin at the site to numb the area.
4. Insert a large-bore intravenous catheter (14-gauge), needle, or any pointy, sharp object that is available (the object should not be wider than a pencil) into the chest just above the third rib in line with the middle of the collarbone and the nipple. The middle of the collarbone is midway between the top of the shoulder and the end of the collarbone near the windpipe. If you hit the rib, move the needle or pointy object upward slightly until it passes over the top of the rib, thus avoiding the blood vessels that course along the bottom of every rib. A gush of air will signal that you have entered the correct space and that you should not push the object in any farther. This will convert the tension pneumothorax from air locked in the chest into an open pneumothorax, where the air can escape.
5. Leave the object in place and put the cutout finger portion of a rubber glove with a slit cut into the end over the opening to create a one-way flutter valve that allows air out but not in.
6. Anchor the object to the chest wall with tape so that it cannot be pulled out or forced farther into the chest.
7. If a hole was made with a knife, monitor the person closely, and if signs of tension redevelop, repeat the procedure above.

How to Put On Surgical Gloves

Putting on surgical gloves is not difficult, but it does require planning and forethought, or you'll easily compromise the gloves' sterility in the process. To don the gloves, follow these steps (for right-handed persons):

1. Wash and thoroughly dry your hands. Prepare a flat surface on which to open the sterile gloves.
2. Carefully open the inner package and expose the gloves without touching them. Avoid contact with the inner surface of the package in order to maintain sterility. The gloves will be marked "left" and "right."
3. Pick up the right glove with your left hand at the folded cuff and carefully slide your right hand into the fingers. Pick up the left glove with the right gloved hand by sliding the four fingers (not the thumb) between the folded cuff and the palm of the glove, then slowly insert the left hand. Adjust and pull up the cuffs without touching exposed skin.
4. Both hands are now in sterile gloves, and the package that contained the gloves can be left open and undisturbed to be used as a sterile field for sterile instruments.

Open (Sucking) Chest Wound

If an object such as a stingray tail, speargun point, marlinspike, or knife enters the chest, a wound that opens into the lung can develop. A sucking sound can often be heard as air passes in and out through the wound each time the person breathes.

Signs and Symptoms
- Painful and difficult breathing
- A sucking sound each time the person breathes
- Bubbles seen at the wound site when the person exhales
- Bubbles of air felt and heard (crackling) on touching the chest wall near the injury
- Signs of a tension pneumothorax

Treatment

1. Seal the opening immediately with any airtight substance (piece of rubber, aluminum foil, plastic bag) and cover it with a 10 x 10-cm (4 x 4-inch) gauze pad, taping it on three sides. (Taping three edges produces a flutter-valve effect.) When the person inhales, the free edge will seal against the skin. As the person exhales, the free edge will allow air in the chest cavity to escape.
2. If an object is stuck in the chest, do not remove it. Place airtight material next to the skin around it, and stabilize it with bulky dressings or pads. Several layers of dressings, clothing, or handkerchiefs placed on the sides of the object will help stabilize it.

Note: A person with an open chest wound below the nipple line may also have an injury to an abdominal organ, such as the spleen or liver.

 ## Weiss Advice

Dressing an Open Chest Wound

An airtight dressing can be improvised from a 10 x 10-cm (4 x 4-inch) gauze pad impregnated with petroleum jelly, honey, or antibiotic ointment. Plastic wrap or some other clean plastic will also work. Tape the dressing in place on three sides only.

ABDOMINAL (BELLY) INJURIES

Abdominal organs are either solid or hollow. When solid organs, such as the spleen or liver, are injured, they bleed internally. Hollow organs can rupture and drain their contents into the abdominal and pelvic cavities, producing a painful and serious inflammatory reaction and infection.

Table 1: Abdominal Organs

Organ	Type	Location
Liver	Solid	RUQ
Stomach	Hollow	RUQ
Spleen	Solid	LUQ
Pancreas	Solid	LUQ
Small and large intestines	Hollow	All quadrants
Kidneys	Solid	Flanks

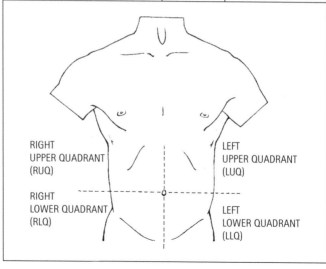

RIGHT UPPER QUADRANT (RUQ)

LEFT UPPER QUADRANT (LUQ)

RIGHT LOWER QUADRANT (RLQ)

LEFT LOWER QUADRANT (LLQ)

Blunt Abdominal Injuries

A blow to the belly from a fall or collision with another object can result in internal organ injuries and bleeding, even though nothing penetrates the skin. Examine the abdomen by pressing on it gently with the tips of your fingers sequentially in all four quadrants. Push slowly and observe for pain, muscle spasms, or rigidity. Normal abdomens are soft and not painful to touch.

Signs and Symptoms

- Signs of shock (weak, rapid pulse; rapid breathing; fear; pale and moist skin; confusion)
- Pain that is at first mild and then becomes severe
- Distention (bloating) of the abdomen
- Pain or rigidity (tightness or hardness) of the belly muscles when pressing in on the abdomen
- Pain referred to the left or right shoulder tip (may indicate a ruptured spleen)
- Nausea or repetitive vomiting
- Bloody urine
- Pain in the abdomen with body movement
- Fever, often with shaking chills

Treatment

1. Evacuate the person to a medical facility as soon as possible.
2. Anticipate and treat for shock.
3. Do not allow the person to eat. If the person is not vomiting, offer small sips of water.

GUNSHOT WOUNDS AND ARROW AND SPEARGUN INJURIES

Gunshot Wounds

Injuries caused by guns differ in severity and type according to velocity of the bullet, power of the gun, whether fragmentation occurs, presence of powder burns, and type of tissue struck. A gunshot wound may cause severe internal damage and bleeding that is not readily visible or apparent. Although the entrance or exit wound may appear small, the damage inside the body may be great. Any person who has suffered a gunshot wound should be evacuated to a medical facility, no matter how minor the external appearance.

Treatment

1. Follow the basic principles of resuscitation, including airway, breathing, circulation, control of bleeding, immobilization of any broken extremities, wound care, and stabilization of the person for transport (see "The ABCs of Marine First Aid: The Primary Survey," page 15).
2. Remove the weapon from where you are giving medical care, remove the ammunition, and open the firing chamber.
3. Provide immediate relief of a tension pneumothorax with pleural decompression.
4. Treat any sucking chest wound with petrolatum-impregnated gauze.
5. Control external bleeding with direct pressure and compression wraps.
6. Treat for shock and hypothermia.
7. Monitor the neurovascular status of an extremity wound; keep the extremity elevated to minimize swelling.
8. Be aware that the path of the bullet cannot be determined by connecting the entrance and exit wounds.
9. For powder burns, remove as much of the powder residue as possible with a scrub brush, because the powder will tattoo the skin if left in place.
10. Expect internal bleeding.

Arrow and Speargun Injuries

Arrowheads and spearguns inflict injury by cutting tissue and blood vessels, causing bleeding and shock.

Treatment

1. Follow the same treatment recommendations as for a gunshot wound.
2. Stabilize the person for transport, leaving any embedded arrow or spear in place during transport if possible. Cut the shaft of the

arrow or spear and leave about 10 cm (4 inches) protruding from the wound to make transport easier. Use rigging cutters to cut the metal shaft of a spear.

3. Fix the portion that remains in the wound with a stack of gauze pads or with cloth and tape.

4. Transfer the person to a medical care facility for removal of the arrow or spear under controlled conditions.

Do Not Remove Embedded Foreign Objects

If a foreign object (such as a knife, spear, or arrow) becomes deeply embedded (impaled) in the body, do not attempt to remove it, because the internal portion may be up against or in a vital organ and acting as a plug, thus preventing further bleeding. Any attempt to remove the object may cause further bleeding and injury. This is particularly true with a hunting (broadhead) arrow.

Instead, pad and bandage the wound around the object and secure it in place with tape. The portion of the object that is sticking out of the wound may be cut to a shorter length to facilitate splinting and transport of the person.

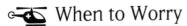 # When to Worry

Internal Bleeding

If bleeding is internal (inside the body), such as from an injured spleen or liver, bleeding ulcer, broken bone, or torn internal blood vessel, the person may suffer from shock. The signs of internal bleeding are the same as those of external bleeding, except that you don't see the blood. They include rapid heartbeat, low blood pressure, shortness of breath, weakness, pale skin color, cool and clammy skin, and confusion. The belly feels firm to the touch, looks distended, and is painful. Blood may be present in the vomit, urine, or stool. Because it is difficult to gauge the rate and severity of internal bleeding, the person requires evacuation to a medical facility.

MUSCLE, LIGAMENT, AND SKELETAL INJURIES

Sprains

A sprain is the stretching or tearing of ligaments, which attach one bone to another. Ligaments are sprained when a joint is twisted or stretched beyond its normal range of motion. Most sprains occur in the ankle and knee.

Signs and Symptoms

Symptoms include tenderness at the site, swelling, bruising, and pain with movement. Because these symptoms are also present with a fracture, it may be difficult to differentiate between the two. If the person can bear weight on the injured ankle or knee, and there is no angular deformity, the injury is likely to be a sprain and not a fracture.

Treatment

First aid for sprains is primarily damage control and summarized by the acronym RICES (rest, ice, compression, elevation, and stabilization). RICES should be maintained for the first 72 hours after any injury. Too often this is prematurely discontinued after only a few hours.

SHOULDER SPICA TO SUPPORT THE ARM AND SHOULDER

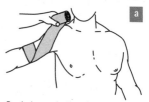

Begin by encircling the upper arm with wide (6-inch is best) elastic bandage and continue upward to the armpit. Continue the wrap around the shoulder.

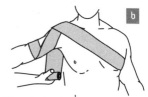

Wrap the bandage across the chest and under the opposite shoulder, through the armpit, and around the back to the injured shoulder.

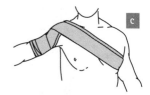

Repeat the pattern as the length of the bandage allows and finish on the upper arm.

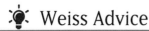 Weiss Advice

RICES FOR SPRAINS AND STRAINS

REST: Resting takes the stress off the injured joint and prevents further damage.

ICE: Ice reduces swelling and eases pain. For ice or cold therapy to be effective, it must be applied early after the injury, and for up to 20 minutes at least three to four times a day, followed by compression bandaging. If a compression wrap is not applied after ice therapy, the joint will swell as soon as the ice is removed. On a cruising boat, where ice may be in short supply, use a package of frozen vegetables as an ice pack and refreeze it for repeated use. Cold river water or seawater can be used if ice is not available. Fill a plastic bag and refill it frequently.

COMPRESSION: Compression wraps prevent swelling and provide some support. One can be made by placing some padding (e.g., socks, gloves, pieces of Ensolite pad) over the sprained joint and then wrapping it with an elastic wrap bandage. Begin the wrap toward the end of the extremity and move upward. For example, with an ankle sprain, start from the toes and move up the foot and over the ankle with the wrap. The wrap should be comfortably tight. If the person experiences numbness, tingling, or increased pain, the compression wrap may be too tight and should be loosened.

ELEVATION: Elevate the injured joint above the level of the heart as much as possible to reduce swelling.

STABILIZATION: Tape or splint the injured part to prevent further injury (see "Weiss Advice: Ankle Support Using a SAM Splint," page 78).

Administer a nonsteroidal anti-inflammatory medication such as ibuprofen (Advil, Motrin) 400–600 mg three times a day (with food) to reduce both pain and inflammation. Depending on the extent of injury, it is usually beneficial to begin mobilization and pain-free activity after 3 to 4 days.

Decreasing pain, tenderness, and swelling, together with increasing stability upon weight bearing, are reassuring signs that the injury is probably a sprain and not a fracture. If the person is not improving,

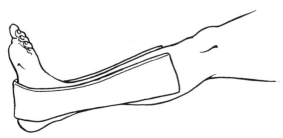

Fig. 28 *Foot or ankle splint*

continue treatment, avoid weight bearing and stress on the injured joint, and seek medical consultation. Even if the "sprain" is in fact a stable fracture, it is not a medical emergency (see "Fractures," page 87).

Ankle Sprain

Sprained ankles are common injuries for boaters. Most commonly, the ligaments on the outside of the joint are injured from rolling the foot inward (inversion) while walking or jumping on an uneven or slippery surface. Ankle sprains frequently occur among paddlers walking over slippery rocks and mud on a riverbank. Kayakers are also prone to ankle injury when the bow of a kayak hits an obstruction. (The new foam bulkheads serving as footrests may help prevent this.) Wet and slippery companionway ladders and decks are common sources of ankle injury aboard watercraft.

Signs and Symptoms

An ankle sprain is the stretching or tearing of ankle ligaments, which attach one bone to another. Ligaments are sprained when the ankle joint is twisted or stretched beyond its normal range of motion.

Treatment

1. First aid begins with RICES (see page 75).
2. If you cannot bear weight at all, you'll have to splint the foot and ankle (**Fig. 28**).

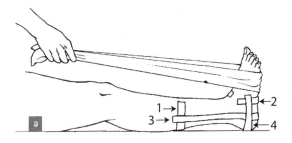

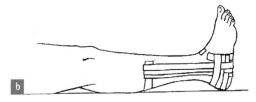

The numbers indicate the order in which the pieces of tape are applied.

Fig. 29 *Sprained ankle taping using a cross-weave stirrup pattern*

3. If you can still walk, the ankle should be taped for support with an open basket cross-weave stirrup pattern to prevent further injury (**Fig. 29**).
   a. Apply an anchor strip halfway around the lower leg about 15 cm (6 inches) above the "bumps" in the ankle. Leave a gap of 4 cm (1.5 inches) between the ends of the tape to allow for swelling.
   b. An additional anchor strip can be applied at the instep of the foot. Leave a 4-cm (1.5-inch) gap between the tape ends.
   c. Apply the first of five stirrup strips. Begin on the inside of the upper anchor, and wrap a piece of tape down the inside of the leg, over the inside bump, across the bottom of the foot, and up the outside part of the leg, over the outside bump, ending at the outer part of the upper anchor.

d. Apply the first of six interconnecting horseshoe strips. Start on the anchor on the inside of the foot, and wrap below the inside bump, around the heel, below the outside bump, ending on the anchor on the outer part of the foot.

e. Repeat steps c and d. Remember to overlap the tape one-half its width. These interlocking strips should provide excellent support when walking. After applying these vertical and horizontal strips, there should be a 2.5- to 5-cm (1- to 2-inch) gap on the top of the foot and ankle, which will allow for any swelling.

f. On both sides, secure the tape ends with two vertical strips of tape running from the foot anchor to the calf anchor.

🔅 Weiss Advice

Ankle Support Using a SAM Splint

Wrap a SAM Splint (**Fig. 30**) around the foot and ankle, with the shoe in place, and secure it with tape. This will help stabilize the joint while walking. You may need to stop periodically to tighten or rewrap the splint.

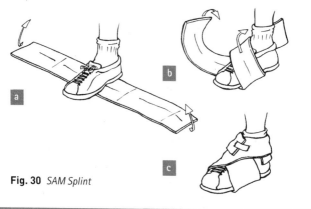

Fig. 30 *SAM Splint*

Sprained or Ruptured Achilles Tendon

Running or walking uphill with a heavy load on the back, or ascending the companionway ladder with a heavy sail, can injure the Achilles tendon, which attaches the calf muscles to the heel. The tendon can rupture completely while running or jumping, in which case it pulls away from the bone or snaps in half.

Signs and Symptoms

If you rupture your Achilles tendon, you'll feel as if someone stabbed the back of your ankle with a sharp object and you'll be unable to bear weight. The person will often hear a snap as the tendon ruptures.

Treatment

If the tendon is strained and not completely torn or ruptured, RICES (see page 75) is the best treatment. Gently stretch the tendon to keep it flexible, and gradually put weight on the foot, then walk as the pain allows. If you rupture your Achilles tendon, walking will not be possible. The foot and ankle should be splinted (see **Fig. 49**, page 110) at a 90-degree angle and the person evacuated. Surgery is needed to repair the torn tendon.

Knee Sprain

Twisting, rotating, or falling in an awkward position can produce a sprain injury to one of the major ligaments that supports the knee. The collateral ligaments support the sides of the knee, while the anterior and posterior cruciate ligaments support and limit motion in the forward and backward directions. The person may note an audible crack or a pop at the time of injury, followed by immediate pain that soon turns into a dull ache. The ache may subside after a while, and the knee will swell and feel as though it's going to give way when weight is put on it or it is turned to the side.

Knee sprains are divided into three degrees of severity based on the amount of ligament that is torn:

■ *First-degree sprains* produce pain, but no instability when the knee is stressed, which indicates that only a few ligament fibers are torn. Treatment is initially RICES (see page 75), and later physical therapy. Walking can usually be resumed with little or no additional support.

- *Second-degree sprains* produce pain and slight instability when the knee is stressed, and indicate that about half of the ligament fibers are torn. Treatment is the same as for a first-degree sprain, but recovery takes longer and surgery may eventually be required. The person should wear a supportive knee immobilizer while walking (**Fig. 31**).

- *Third-degree sprains* produce significant instability and indicate a completely torn ligament. Initiate treatment with RICES (see page 75), and prohibit walking without a supportive knee immobilizer in place. Even with a third-degree tear, many persons can still walk with some additional sup-

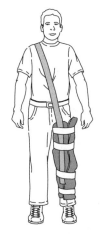

Fig. 31 *Duct-tape suspenders supporting an improvised knee immobilizer*

port. If after applying an improvised knee immobilizer, the knee still feels unstable and prone to buckling with weight, the person should be evacuated without walking.

☀ Weiss Advice

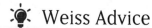

Knee Immobilizer

A knee immobilizer (knee splint) can be improvised from an Ensolite or Therm-a-Rest pad, a foam seat cushion, a life jacket, a newspaper, a firm blanket, sail battens, tent poles, internal pack frame stays, or clothing held together with tape or bandannas. The immobilizer should be cylindrical and extend from mid-thigh down to mid-calf. If possible, cut out a circular hole for the kneecap. Duct tape can be used to fashion suspenders to prevent the knee immobilizer from slipping downward while walking (**Fig. 31**).

Torn Knee Cartilage (Meniscus)

The meniscus acts as a shock absorber for the knee and rests between the thigh and shin bones (tibia and fibula). Partial and total tears of the meniscus often occur at the same time that ligaments are torn.

Signs and Symptoms

Pain, localized to one side of the knee joint and made worse by walking, is the most common symptom. Clicking or locking of the knee may be present. Occasionally, the joint can become locked in a partially flexed and painful position, and the person will not be able to move the knee.

Treatment

1. Treatment is rest, ice, and ibuprofen (Advil, Motrin) 400 mg three times a day with food.
2. If the knee feels unstable, wrap a protective immobilizer around it (see **Fig. 31**).
3. If the person has a locked knee, attempt to unlock it by positioning the person with the leg hanging over the edge of a table or flat surface, with the knee in approximately 90 degrees of flexion. After a period for muscle relaxation, apply in-line traction to the leg with inward and outward rotation in an attempt to unlock the joint. Pain medications and muscle relaxers (lorazepam [Ativan]) may facilitate this.

Patellofemoral Syndrome

This common overuse syndrome produces a dull, aching pain under the kneecap or in the center of the knee. The pain is aggravated by climbing or descending hills and by sitting for long periods with the knees bent. This syndrome is one of the most common causes of knee pain in sailing. Repetitive hiking out (extending the upper body to shift weight and balance the boat), kneeling, climbing companionway steps, and twisting exacerbate this condition.

Signs and Symptoms

The knee may be swollen, and crackling sounds can often be heard when the knee is flexed and straightened.

Treatment

Treatment is rest, ice, and anti-inflammatory medication such as ibuprofen (Advil, Motrin) 400 mg three times a day with food. A patella tendon band placed around the leg, below the kneecap, may help prevent pain during walking (see "Weiss Advice: Patella Tendon Band" below). Use of two trekking poles while walking will help absorb impact on the knees.

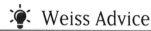

☀ Weiss Advice

Patella Tendon Band

To improvise a patella tendon band, roll a bandanna or triangular bandage tightly along its long axis. Wrap this around the leg just below the kneecap, then tie it securely.

Strains

A strain is an injury to a muscle or its tendon. The tendon connects the muscle to the bone. Strains often result from overexertion, or lifting and pulling a heavy object without good body mechanics. Strains, especially back strains, can sometimes be disabling.

Prevention

Paddlers frequently experience injury from overuse of the muscles and tendons of the wrist, forearm, elbow, and shoulder. Prevent injury by stretching, loosening your paddle grip, and changing hand positions. Adjust hands on the paddle shaft to shoulder width in order to engage the shoulders and reduce wrist strain. Modification of paddling techniques and the boats' outfitting, choice of paddles, and proper stretching before and after exercise are the most important measures for preventing strains.

Signs and Symptoms

Symptoms are the same as for sprains. Muscle spasms often accompany a strain injury and can be very painful.

Treatment

Muscle relaxers such as lorazepam (Ativan) may be helpful in relieving spasms, but they also produce drowsiness and impair coordination.

As a guideline, the following times are required for initial healing of the musculoskeletal system:

- Muscles: 6 to 8 weeks
- Bones: 6 to 12 weeks
- Tendons and ligaments: 12 to 36 weeks (some ligaments may take 12 months or longer to heal)

Carpal Tunnel Syndrome

Offshore helmspeople and paddlers are susceptible to this hand and wrist injury, which arises from tightly gripping the wheel, tiller, or paddle for extended periods. The carpal tunnel ligament, which crosses the underside of the wrist like a watchband, becomes tight and compresses the underlying nerves to the hand.

Signs and Symptoms

Tingling and numbness in the first three fingers and part of the fourth finger, and accompanying hand weakness, result from compression of the underlying nerves.

Treatment

Treatment includes RICES (see page 75) and anti-inflammatory medication such as ibuprofen (Advil, Motrin) 600 mg three times daily with food. During activity, a wrist brace can be made with an ACE bandage around both the wrist and hand (to limit motion of the wrist), and a splint (similar to one used for hand fractures) can be used at night. Cock the hand up about 30 degrees, in the position of function.

Back Strain

Back pain ranks among the top ten most common ailments in backpackers, sailors, and paddlers. Sailors frequently suffer lower back injury while hauling sails from lockers onto the deck, raising heavy sails, pulling up the anchor, and cranking on winches. Back and neck pain are common among windsurfers, particularly among those who up haul the rig (as opposed to water starting). Dinghy racers are at risk while hiking out (extending the upper body) to shift weight and balance the boat. Scuba divers injure their back when putting on their buoyancy compensator (BC) vests with heavy tanks, or walking with heavy gear. The repetitive motion of hand-paddling a surfboard in a prone position for long periods commonly results in shoulder, neck, and back strain. The lower part of the back, the lumbar spine, holds most of the weight of the body and is, therefore, most susceptible to problems.

Prevention

Preventing a back injury is a lot easier than trying to recover from one. While on the trail or engaging in water sports, you can do several things to lessen the chances of injuring your back.

- Stretch before lifting and paddling, especially in the morning when your muscles are cold and stiff.
- When putting on a heavy pack, keep your back straight and in a neutral position. Slide your pack onto one thigh and slip one shoulder into a loosened shoulder strap. Roll the pack onto your back and use your legs, not your back and arms, to lift yourself up.
- When lifting, always keep objects close to the body, not at arm's length, which increases spinal stress seven to ten times (a 1-kg [2-pound] weight held away from the body exacts the same stress on your spine as a 9-kg [20-pound] weight held close). Scuba divers should carry tanks in both arms across the chest to prevent unbalanced back stress and injury.
- Adjust the pack so that as much weight as possible is on the hip belt instead of the shoulder straps.
- Use a walking stick for added balance and support.
- Learn how to break out a set anchor using the boat's engine and motion in waves. Use an anchor windlass for heavy anchors.
- Position sails belowdecks for easy access during sail changes.

- Plan to change sails before storms and rough seas develop.
- Pay attention to body mechanics when lifting heavy objects or engaging in repetitive movements that involve the lower back. Face the object being lifted; keep it close to your body, and use the muscles of the legs, buttocks, and hips to do the work.
- Scuba divers should not put on a BC vest and tank like an overcoat; put both arms into the BC (while someone is holding it or with it resting in a bench rack), then settle it on both shoulders before bearing the weight. Bend from the knees when lifting, not from the waist. Be aware of spinal alignment, and proceed slowly and carefully when climbing the ladder to reboard the boat. Take off your gear (BC vest with tank and weights) in the water, then pass it to someone on the stern deck.

Signs and Symptoms

The symptoms include pain and muscle spasm across the middle of the lower back. Although back pain may be a symptom of a more serious condition, it is often due to strained muscles.

Treatment

If possible, rest on your back with a pillow under your knees or on your side with a pillow between your legs for 1 to 2 days before resuming gentle and graded activity. Extended bed rest and inactivity can actually weaken the back and delay recovery. Most people with sudden back pain will recover completely within 2 to 4 weeks.

Other Treatments

1. Anti-inflammatory medication, such as ibuprofen (Advil, Motrin) 600 mg three times a day (with food) for 5 to 7 days
2. Application of cold compresses
3. Gentle massage
4. Muscle relaxers, such as lorazepam (Ativan), to relieve muscle spasms

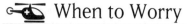 # When to Worry

Back Pain

If back pain is severe and not made worse with movement or change in position, it may be due to some other serious internal problem, such as an aortic aneurysm (bulging of the aorta) or kidney stone or infection, which can cause the pain to radiate to the back. If pain is severe, obtain medical consultation as soon as possible. Also seek medical attention if you experience shooting pains or tingling down the leg, loss of sensation in your arms or legs, problems with bowel or bladder function, or leg or foot weakness, which are all signs of spinal nerve compression.

OVERUSE INJURIES

Rotator Cuff Tendonitis

This painful shoulder injury results from the repetitive motion (overuse) involved in sailing, paddling, surfboarding, and other water sports. Kayakers are prone to overuse shoulder injuries from playing in river hydraulics (where the water flows back on itself). Improper techniques may sometimes be a contributing factor.

Signs and Symptoms

Symptoms include shoulder pain that worsens with overhead arm movement, and diminished flexibility and strength in the shoulder and arm.

Treatment

Avoid aggravating the injury with the same motions that caused it. Begin RICES treatment (see page 75) and anti-inflammatory drugs. Physical therapy, with exercises to increase flexibility, strength, and range of motion, can help restore balance to the shoulder muscles.

Cervical Spine Strain

Known as "sail trimmer's neck," this injury occurs in sailors who constantly look up to the sails and masthead.

Signs and Symptoms

Over time, numbness and tingling shooting down the arm may result from a pinched nerve in the cervical (neck) spine.

Treatment

In addition to RICES (see page 75), anti-inflammatory medication and muscle relaxants can be useful. The neck muscles and ligaments may benefit from gentle cervical traction and support with a large rolled-up towel wrapped around the neck and folded under the chin to support the head and limit movement. A life jacket can be fitted with duct tape to offer this support.

FRACTURES

A fracture is any break or crack in a bone. An open, or compound, fracture occurs when the overlying skin at the fracture site has been punctured or cut. The bone is in direct contact with the world outside the body. This happens when a sharp bone end protrudes through the skin or from a direct blow that breaks the skin as it fractures the bone. The bone may or may not be visible in the wound.

A closed fracture is one in which there is no wound on the skin anywhere near the fracture site. A closed fracture can become an open fracture if it is not treated correctly.

Open fractures are more likely than closed ones to produce significant blood loss. The bone is contaminated by being exposed to the environment and usually becomes infected. An infected bone is very difficult to treat and causes long-term problems.

How to Tell If a Bone Is Fractured

It may be difficult to differentiate a fractured bone from a sprained ligament or bruised bone. When in doubt, splint the extremity and assume it is fractured. Sometimes, an X-ray is needed to make a proper diagnosis.

Signs of a Possible Fracture

- *Deformity.* The limb appears to be in an unnatural position. Compare the injured limb with the uninjured limb on the opposite side. Look for differences in length, angle, and rotation.
- *Pain and tenderness* are felt over a specific point (point tenderness).
- *Inability to use the extremity.* For example, someone who twists

an ankle and is unable to bear weight should be suspected of having a broken ankle rather than a sprained ankle.

- *Rapid swelling and bruising* (black-and-blue discoloration) are apparent.
- *Crepitus (grating).* A grinding sensation can sometimes be felt and heard when touching or moving a fractured limb.
- *Inappropriate motion.* Motion at a point in a limb where no joint exists indicates a fracture.

Treatment: General Guidelines

1. Inspect the site of injury for any deformity, angulation, or damage to the skin. Cut away the clothing at the fracture site with blunt-tipped scissors. This will prevent excess movement of the injured area and help protect the person from the environment.
2. Stop any bleeding with direct pressure.
3. Check the circulation below the fracture site by feeling for pulses and inspecting the skin for abnormal color changes. Pallor (paleness), bluish discoloration, or a colder hand or foot compared with the noninjured side may indicate a damaged blood vessel. Without circulation, a limb can survive for only about 6 to 8 hours. Check sensation by using a safety pin or pointed object to determine if the sharp sensation is felt equally on both extremities.
4. Because of the force necessary to break a bone, any person with a fracture should be examined carefully for other injuries.
5. Splint all fractures before the person is moved, unless the location presents an immediate danger to the person. Splinting prevents movement of broken bones, which avoids additional injury to bones, muscles, nerves, and blood vessels. Splinting also reduces pain, prevents a closed fracture from becoming open, and makes evacuating the person easier.

Treatment of Open Fractures

1. *Clean.* Irrigate the wound with very large amounts (1–3 L [1–3 quarts]) of sterile saline or disinfected water to remove any obvious dirt. Use a syringe and 18-gauge catheter (see "Cleaning Wounds," page 122).

2. *Dress.* After thoroughly cleansing the wound and bone, cover it with a sterile dressing. Leave the dressing in place; frequent inspections of the wound increases the chance of infection.

3. *Reduce.* Try to realign (straighten) the extremity to its normal position to facilitate splinting. Don't worry if the bone is pushed back under the skin, as this is better than leaving it exposed. To realign the broken bone, pull gently on the limb below the fracture site, in a direction that straightens it, while someone else holds counter-traction on the limb above the fracture. While continuing to hold traction, immediately apply a splint to prevent further motion and damage. Discontinue traction if pain or resistance increases significantly. (See "Treatment of Closed Fractures," page 90.)

4. *Splint.* In general, a splint should be long enough to incorporate the joints above and below the fracture. This prevents the muscles and tendons from moving sections of the fractured bone. A 10 x 91-cm (4 x 36-inch) foam-padded aluminum splint works best.

5. *Antibiotics:* Because all open fracture wounds are contaminated, start antibiotics such as cephalexin (Keflex) or levofloxacin (Levaquin). Infection progresses with the time to definitive treatment (i.e., operating room). Evacuation as soon as possible is always indicated.

Splinting

For joint fractures, immobilize the long bones above and below the joint. The splint should be rigid, well-padded, and multidimensional, with splint materials on two or more sides of the injured part. The splint should immobilize the fractured part in a position of function. Functional position means that the leg is almost straight with a slight flexion at the knee (place a rolled-up towel behind the knee), the ankle and elbow are bent at 90 degrees, the wrist is straight or slightly extended, and the fingers are flexed in a curve, as if to hold a can of soda or a baseball.

■ Remove all jewelry, such as watches, bracelets, and rings, from the person before applying the splint.

■ Use plenty of padding, especially at the bony protrusions of the wrist, elbow, ankle, and knees, but keep the splint appropriate in size and bulk. It should be comfortable, compact, and not cumbersome. If necessary, keep the padding dry by covering the splint with a plastic bag; check for moisture frequently, and change the padding if it becomes wet.

▪ Secure the splint in place with strips of clothing, belts, pieces of rope, webbing, pack straps, elastic wrap bandages, or duct tape.

▪ Fashion the splint on the uninjured body part first and then transfer it to the injured area to minimize discomfort.

▪ Elevate the injured body part as much as possible after splinting to minimize swelling.

▪ Always check the circulation after applying a splint or after any manipulation. Check the pulse in the foot or wrist, skin color, and temperature often to make certain that swelling inside the splint has not cut off circulation.

▪ Monitor sensation: numbness, tingling, and increased pain may also be a sign of swelling that increases over time.

▪ Administer pain medication.

▪ Improvisation is often necessary. Splints can be fashioned from a variety of materials on a boat, including foam cushions, sail battens, spears, fishing poles, telescoping poles, life vests, paddles, and more. A scuba diver's buoyancy vest or an inflatable life vest can work as a temporary inflatable splint when bound with an elastic wrap bandage or duct tape. Simply use the oral inflation tube to achieve the correct dimensions and tension. The padded-aluminum SAM Splint is ideally suited for the marine environment. Its versatility makes it useful for a variety of injuries and fractures; it is waterproof and reusable.

Treatment of Closed Fractures

In general, realignment of a fractured limb to a normal anatomical position is preferred, especially if the circulation to the extremity is impaired or gross deformity prevents splinting and evacuation. Alignment of a long bone reduces pain and bleeding at the fracture site, and may allow for limited function. Realignment is easier if it is done early, before swelling, muscle spasm, and pain make it more difficult (see **Fig. 32**).

1. Pull gently on the limb below the fracture site in a direction that straightens it, while someone else holds counter-traction on the

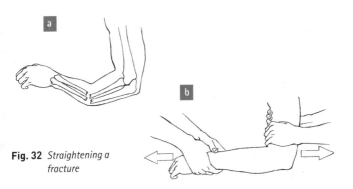

Fig. 32 *Straightening a fracture*

limb above the fracture. Discontinue the maneuver if the person complains of a significant increase in pain, or if resistance is met.

2. After the limb has been straightened, immediately apply a splint before releasing traction. If alignment cannot be achieved, splint the extremity as it lies.

3. After any manipulation, recheck to see whether circulation has been restored or improved.

4. Joint fractures are generally splinted in the position the joint is in at the time of injury; if the circulation is impaired, or there is loss of sensation beyond the fracture site indicating nerve compression and injury, try to bring the joint into a neutral anatomic position before splinting.

Neck and Spine Fractures

Fractures of the neck and spine can damage the spinal cord and lead to permanent paralysis. Any accident that places excessive force or pressure on the head, neck, or back, such as a fall, head injury, or diving accident, can also result in a fracture of the spine.

The decision to initiate and to maintain spine immobilization in the wilderness or at sea has significant ramifications. An otherwise ambulatory person, or one who could remain on a boat, would require a potentially expensive, hazardous, and arduous rescue. The added delay could worsen other injuries and predispose the person and the rest of the party to hypothermia or other environmental hazards. Although in general it is always better to err on the side of being overprotective, everyone with a bump or cut on the head does not need to have the spine immobilized. With training and experience, one can learn to confidently perform a spine examination that can distinguish between an uninjured and possibly injured spine. This is an important part of the curriculum in wilderness medical training courses. Always consider the mechanism of injury (e.g., a surfer plunging head first into shallow water from the top of a wave or a crew member hit in the head with a swinging boom) when evaluating a possible spinal injury.

Treatment

If a spine injury is suspected, the medic should immobilize the head, neck, and trunk to prevent any movement. If the person is lying in a dangerous location and must be moved quickly, the head and neck should be held firmly by one medic's hands, while as many people as available place their arms under the person from either side. The medic at the head says, "Ready, go," and with everyone lifting simultaneously, the person is lifted as a unit and moved to a safer location. After the person is moved, one medic should continue to hold the head firmly with two hands until the spine is immobilized.

If the neck lies at an angle to the body, control the weight of the person's head by using a firm grip while you align the head and neck in one steady and continuous motion with gentle in-line traction. Avoid a forceful pull on the neck. A second medic should then place a cervical collar around the neck to provide some stability.

Cervical collars alone do not provide adequate immobilization. After a collar is placed around the neck, plastic bags, stuff sacks, a life jacket, socks filled with sand, or rolled-up towels and clothing should be placed on either side of the head and neck, and secured to the head with tape or straps to prevent any side-to-side movement. The rest of the body should then be secured to a flat board to prevent any movement. If the person needs to be turned onto their side because of vomiting, maintain spine precautions by logrolling the person (see **Fig. 33**).

Logrolling a Person with Multiple Rescuers

If the person is vomiting or must be rolled or turned to place insulation underneath, logroll the person with the head and body held as a unit (**Fig. 33**). In the event of a suspected spine injury, it is generally better to send for professional rescue assistance rather than attempt to transport the person yourself.

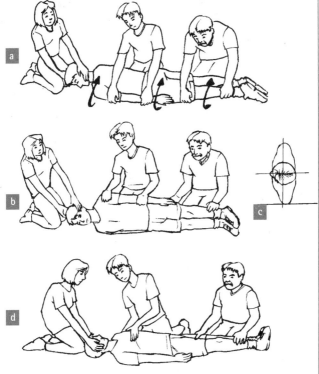

Fig. 33 *Logrolling a victim with multiple rescuers*

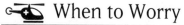 # When to Worry

Spinal Injury

Suspect a spinal injury, and initiate and maintain spine immobilization, after trauma that involves the head, neck, or back when:

- The person is unconscious.
- The person feels pain in the back of the neck or the middle of the back, or experiences discomfort when those areas are touched.
- There is numbness, tingling, or diminished sensation in any part of an arm or leg.
- There is weakness or inability to move the arms, legs, hands, or feet.
- A person has an altered level of consciousness (see "Head Injuries," page 46) or is under the influence of drugs or alcohol (under these circumstances, the exam is not reliable).
- A very painful injury, such as a femur or pelvic fracture, dislocated shoulder, or broken rib, may distract the person from noticing neck pain.

☀ Weiss Advice

Improvised Cervical Collars

A cervical collar can be improvised by using a SAM Splint, sleeping pad, newspaper, backpack hip belt, fanny pack, sleeping pad, life jacket, or clothing.

SAM Splint Cervical Collar

Create a bend in the SAM Splint approximately 15 cm (6 inches) from the end of the splint. This bend will form the front support that holds the chin. Place the front support underneath the chin and wrap the remainder of the splint around the neck. Create side supports by squeezing together the slack in the splint to form flares under each ear. Finally, squeeze the back of the splint in a similar manner to create a back support, then secure the whole thing with tape.

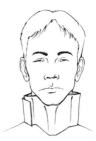

SAM Splint cervical collar

Sleeping Pad Collar

Fold the pad lengthwise into thirds, and center it over the back of the person's neck. Wrap the pad around the neck, under the chin, and secure it in place with tape.

If the pad is not long enough, extensions can be taped or tied on. Blankets, beach towels, or even a rolled-up plastic tarp can be used in a similar fashion.

Padded Hip Belt Collar

A padded hip belt removed from a large internal or external frame backpack can sometimes be modified to function as a cervical collar. If the belt is too long, overlap the ends and secure them with duct tape.

Clothing Collar

Any bulky item of clothing can be used. Wrap a wide elastic wrap bandage around the entire item first, to compress the material and to make it more rigid and supportive before placing it on the neck.

Jaw Fractures

Signs and Symptoms

A fracture of the mandible (jawbone) should be suspected when pain and swelling are present at the site, the person is unable to open or close the mouth as usual, or the teeth do not fit together in a normal fashion.

Treatment

Apply ice to the site to reduce swelling and pain. A liquid diet should be maintained until the person reaches the hospital.

Facial Fractures

Signs and Symptoms

- Tenderness is felt in response to touching the cheekbones or bones around the eyes, with swelling and black-and-blue discoloration of the skin.
- Abnormal movement of the upper face when you grasp the upper teeth between your thumb and forefinger and gently rock the teeth back and forth.
- The person may have double vision, especially when looking upward.
- The fractured side of the face may feel numb.

Treatment

Elevate the person's head and apply ice to reduce swelling. Evacuate the person to a medical facility.

Collarbone (Clavicle) Fractures

These most likely occur from a fall directly onto the shoulder.

Signs and Symptoms

The person usually holds the fractured arm against the chest wall for support, to prevent motion of the broken bone. Swelling and tenderness are present at the site.

Treatment

Splint the arm against the chest with a sling and swath, or with safety pins while utilizing the sleeved portion of the shirt or jacket to pin the arm to the chest part of the garment (**Fig. 34**). Whenever the arm is immobilized in this way, a life jacket should be refit to the person and be worn whenever practical. Self-inflating oral tubes and manually activated inflators should be readily accessible.

☀ Weiss Advice

Making a Sling with Safety Pins

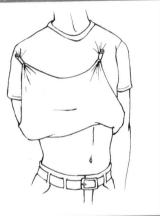

If the person is wearing a long-sleeved shirt or jacket, pin the injured arm to the chest portion of the garment with two safety pins. If the person is wearing a short-sleeved shirt, fold the bottom of the shirt up and over the injured arm to create a pouch. Pin the pouch to the sleeve and chest section of the shirt to immobilize the arm.

Fig. 34 *Shoulder immobilizer using the victim's own shirt and two safety pins*

Shoulder and Upper Arm (Humerus) Fractures

Signs and Symptoms

There is usually pain and tenderness at the site and inability to use the arm. Unlike shoulder dislocations, persons with a fracture will still be able to bring the injured arm in tightly and comfortably against the chest and touch their opposite shoulder with the hand of the injured arm.

Treatment

Upper arm fractures should be immobilized with a well-padded splint, which extends from the armpit down the inner part of the arm, around the elbow, and back up the outside of the arm to the shoulder. After splinting, secure the arm against the body using a sling and swath, or safety pins (**Fig. 34**, page 97). The elbow should be flexed less than 90 degrees to avoid pinching off any blood vessels.

Elbow, Forearm, and Wrist Fractures
These usually occur after a fall on an outstretched hand.

Signs and Symptoms
A broken wrist sometimes has a deformity that makes it look like an upside-down fork.

Treatment
1. If there is an obvious deformity and circulation has been cut off to the hand (there is no pulse at the wrist, and the hand is turning blue and cold compared with the uninjured hand), apply firm traction to straighten the deformity.
2. A splint for a wrist, forearm, or elbow fracture should include both the elbow and hand. Apply a well-padded, U-shaped splint that extends from the hand to the elbow on both sides and wraps around the elbow like a sandwich. The elbow should be bent at 90 degrees, the wrist should be as straight as possible, and the hand should be in a position of function with the fingers curled around something soft, such as a rolled-up glove, sock, or bandage (**Fig. 35**).
3. After splinting, secure the arm against the body for added support.

☀ Weiss Advice

The SAM Splint for Arms

The SAM Splint, a versatile and lightweight padded-aluminum splint, is excellent for splinting upper extremity fractures. It changes from flexible to rigid when bent into a U-shape down its long axis. The SAM Splint can be used for splinting arms in almost any position. The blue side of the splint, slightly thicker and softer than the orange side, should be placed against the skin.

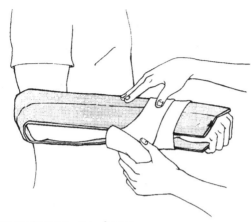

Fig. 35 *SAM Splint for elbow, forearm,*
or wrist fracture

Hand and Finger Fractures
Prevention
Hand and finger injuries (even amputation) are common aboard sail-boats, occurring most often while trimming sails and handling lines under tension. Know how to use winches properly and how to ease or release lines wrapped around the winch. Wear protective gloves to improve grip, prevent rope burns, and avoid superficial injuries. Keep hands and fingers clear of the space between the winch drum and the line. Use caution and follow safety guidelines when using a power windlass for the anchor chain or an electrically powered winch for adjusting lines. Blunt trauma to fingers (jamming fingers) is also common aboard boats.

Signs and Symptoms
A jammed finger may appear crooked, swollen, and discolored, and may be very painful.

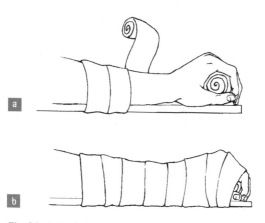

Fig. 36 *Splint for hand fractures, with fingers curled around a roll or bandage*

Treatment

If the finger is not deformed and moves normally at all joints, it should be iced and elevated. After removing rings and bracelets, place a rolled pair of socks or elastic wrap bandage in the palm to keep the fingers curled in a grabbing position (position of function) and secure this in place with an elastic wrap or gauze bandage (**Fig. 36**). Keep the tips of the fingers uncovered in order to check circulation.

Splint a broken finger by buddy-taping the injured finger to an adjacent uninjured finger (**Fig. 37**). Elevate hand injuries to minimize swelling.

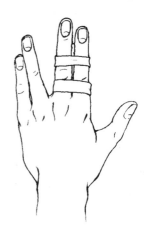

Fig. 37 *Finger splint, with fingers buddy-taped*

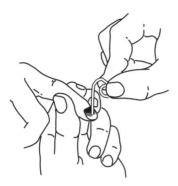

Fig. 38 *Draining a subungual hematoma with a hot paper clip*

Blood Under a Nail (Subungual Hematoma)

A crush injury to a finger (or toe) often causes a painful hematoma (collection of blood) to form under the nail. To relieve the pressure and pain, clean the nail with a 10% povidone-iodine (Betadine) swab, and place the finger on a firm surface. Heat the tip of a paper clip until it glows red hot; place the hot tip of the clip gently onto the nail over the center of the hematoma; as the clip perforates the nail, blood will spurt out and relieve the pressure. This procedure (**Fig. 38**) will not injure the nail bed.

Rib Fractures

See "Chest Injuries: Rib Fractures," page 62.

Pelvic Fractures

Pelvic fractures are devastating injuries, often accompanied by extensive internal bleeding that can be fatal. In addition to losing large amounts of blood into the pelvis from broken bones and torn blood vessels, the person with a pelvic fracture often has other major internal injuries and bleeding. The person can go into shock and bleed to death internally without any sign of external bleeding. Organs such as the bladder or intestines may also be damaged.

Signs and Symptoms

There may be pain in the pelvis, hip, or lower back, and inability to bear weight. Pressing or squeezing gently on the pelvis at or below the beltline will produce pain. If the broken pelvis is unstable, movement of the bones may be felt when compressing the pelvis. If an unstable pelvis is found during assessment, don't do any further exams of the pelvis since further pressing or squeezing of the pelvis can dislodge internal blood clots and cause more bleeding. If the bladder or urethra is damaged, there may be blood at the tip of the penis or in the urine, or the person may be unable to urinate. Follow the instructions for inserting a urinary catheter (see "Urinary Retention and Catheterization of the Urinary Bladder," page 181).

Treatment

Stabilization and compression of the broken pelvis with a pelvic sling or binder will help control bleeding and may save the person's life. It's a technique that works, even for the worst type of pelvic fractures, known as open-book fractures because the pelvic ring has sprung open like the pages of a book. Compression "closes the book," reduces pain, slows bleeding, and promotes clot formation as the person is transported to an emergency department.

The commercially available SAM Pelvic Sling has been developed by SAM Medical Products, the makers of the SAM Splint, for pelvic immobilization and stabilization. On long expeditions and voyages, it should be considered for the medical kit.

Clothes, sheets, an inflatable sleeping pad (**Fig. 39**), or a canvas bosun's chair can be used to improvise a pelvic sling in the backcountry or at sea (**Fig. 40**). First, remove any objects from the person's pockets and remove the belt so that pressure of the sling doesn't cause additional pain by pressing items against the pelvis. Then, slide a sheet, jacket, sleeping pad, or other improvised sling under the person's buttocks and center it under the bony prominences (greater trochanters) at the outer part of the upper thighs or hips. Cross the object over the front of the pelvis and tighten the sling by pulling both ends and securing with a knot, clamp, or duct tape. The sling should be tightened so that it is snug. If an inflatable sleeping pad is used, inflate the pad after securing it to increase the pressure exerted on the pelvis.

Fig. 39

Wrap a Therm-a-Rest or other inflatable sleeping pad around the pelvis and secure it with duct tape. Then blow into the valve and inflate the pad as for sleeping. This will apply circumferential pressure to the broken pelvis.

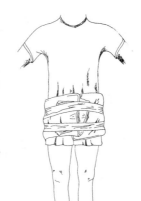

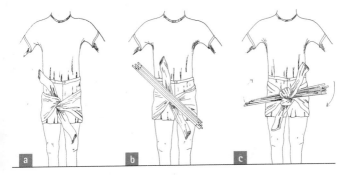

Fig. 40

  a *Slide an article of clothing or sheet or tent fly under the victim's pelvis and center it under the bony prominences at the outer part of the hips. Cross this over the front of the pelvis and tie it together with an overhand knot.*

  b *Place tent poles, a stick, or similar object on the knot and tie another overhand knot.*

  c *Twist the poles or stick until the pelvic sling becomes tight.*

Place padding between the legs and gently tie the legs together to further stabilize the fracture in a position that is most comfortable for the person. Treat for shock, but do not elevate the legs. Arrange for medical evacuation.

Thigh (Femur) Fractures

Signs and Symptoms

A broken femur can produce severe blood loss and lead to shock. When the femur breaks, the thigh muscles spasm, pulling the thigh into a more spherical shape, which allows a greater amount of blood to escape into the surrounding tissues. The broken bone ends overlap and dig into the muscle, causing additional injury, extreme pain, and further blood loss. Often, the broken leg will appear shortened and the foot may be rotated outward, away from the other leg.

Treatment

The best splint for a femur fracture is one that produces traction (see "Weiss Advice: Traction Splint," page 105) to stretch the muscles back to their normal length. This will significantly reduce blood loss, muscle spasms, and pain, and will facilitate evacuation. First, apply traction with your hands by holding the person's foot and pulling the leg back into normal alignment. Try to pull the injured leg out to its normal length, using the uninjured leg as a guide. Once you have started pulling traction, do not release it. If it's just you and the injured person, create the traction splint first, then pull and maintain traction with the device. On a boat, if evacuation is imminent or dangerous sea conditions and weather prevent you from creating the traction splint, bind the injured leg to the good one with wide sail ties or other straps. Good padding is required between the legs and on the outside of the fractured leg when making this "buddy splint." Secure the person's legs effectively in the litter to minimize movement during evacuation.

☀️ Weiss Advice

Traction Splint

A variety of techniques are used for improvising a traction splint with limited materials in the backcountry or on a boat. An improvised traction splint has six components:

- Ankle hitch
- Upper thigh (groin) hitch
- Rigid support that is longer than the leg
- Securing the two hitches to the rigid support
- Producing traction (trucker's hitch)
- Padding

WARNING: Before applying an improvised splint, test your creation on an uninjured person or the uninjured leg of the person.

1. **Apply an ankle hitch.** It is best to leave the shoe or boot on the person's foot and apply the hitch over it. Cut out the toe of the shoe to periodically check the circulation in the foot.

   ■ **Double runner stirrup:** Fold two long, narrow, and strong pieces of material (webbing, triangular bandages, or bandannas folded into cravats; pieces of rope; or even shoelaces) into loops and lay one over and one behind the ankle, making sure the ends of each loop are facing in opposite directions (**Fig. 41**). Pull the ends through the loop on both sides. The

Fig. 41 *Double runner stirrup ankle hitch*

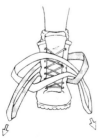

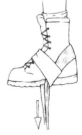

Fig. 42 *Traction in line with the leg*

Continued on next page

Continued from previous page

hitch should fit snugly and flat against the ankle. Adjust the two pieces of material so that the ends are centered under the arch of the shoe and the traction is in line with the leg (**Fig. 42**). The foot should be at a 90-degree angle with the ankle.

■ **S-configuration hitch:** This type of hitch is preferred if the person also has an injury to the foot or ankle, because traction is pulled from the person's calf instead of the ankle. Lay a long piece of webbing or other similar material over the upper part of the ankle (lower calf) in an S-shaped configuration. Wrap both ends of the webbing behind the ankle and up through the loop on the other side. Pull the ends down on either side of the arch of the foot to tighten the hitch, then tie an overhand knot (**Fig. 43**).

■ **Buck's traction:** For extended transports, this system is more comfortable, but must be checked periodically for slippage. Wrap duct tape around a piece of Ensolite, foam, or other material to create a stirrup (**Fig. 44**). Secure the entire unit to the lower leg with an elastic wrap or other improvised bandage. This system greatly increases the surface area over which traction is applied and decreases the potential for painful pressure points and compression of blood vessels leading to the foot.

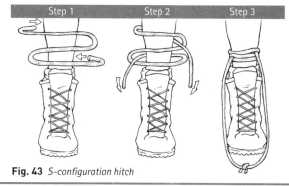

Fig. 43 *S-configuration hitch*

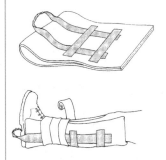

Fig. 44 *Buck's traction*

2. Apply the upper thigh hitch. Tightly wrap a rolled-up jacket or other material (e.g., belt, webbing, fanny pack, or pack straps) around the upper part of the thigh and tie an overhand knot. A rigging harness or climbing harness works well, and paddlers can use an inverted life jacket worn like a diaper. Regardless of the material used, make sure to pad the groin and inner thigh.

3. Apply rigid support to the outside of the injured leg and secure it between the two hitches. Place a rigid, straight object that is at least a foot longer than the leg against the outside of the leg and secure it to the upper thigh hitch with tape or strapping material. You can use one or two poles lashed together with duct tape, a water ski, a boat hook, a mop, tent poles, a canoe or kayak paddle, or a straight tree branch.

Attach the ankle hitch to the rigid support. A blanket pin can be placed in the end of a pole to provide an anchor for the traction system. A Prusik knot (**Fig. 45**) can be used as an attachment point on almost any straight object.

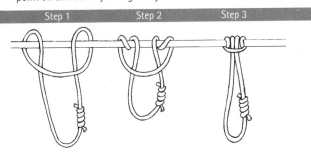

Step 1   Step 2   Step 3

Fig. 45 *Tying a Prusik knot*

Continued on next page

Continued from previous page

4. **Apply traction.** The amount of traction required will vary with the individual. A stopping point for pulling traction is when the injured leg looks to be back to its normal length (compare it

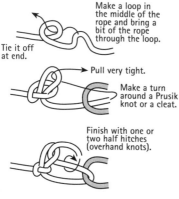

Make a loop in the middle of the rope and bring a bit of the rope through the loop.

Tie it off at end.

Pull very tight.

Make a turn around a Prusik knot or a cleat.

Finish with one or two half hitches (overhand knots).

Fig. 46 *Trucker's hitch*

with the uninjured leg), or when the person is more comfortable. Use a trucker's hitch to gain mechanical advantage when pulling traction (**Fig. 46**).

After applying traction, check the circulation and sensation in the foot every 30 minutes. If the pulse is lost or diminished with traction, or if the foot turns blue or cold, reduce the amount of traction in the splint until the color and pulse return.

5. **Apply padding.** Pad the foot, ankle, and leg at all points where they come into contact with the splint and hitches. Secure the entire splint firmly to the leg (**Fig 47**).

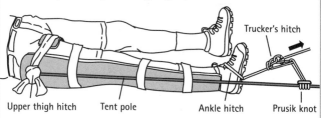

Trucker's hitch

Upper thigh hitch   Tent pole   Ankle hitch   Prusik knot

Fig. 47 *Completed femoral traction splint with Prusik knot used as an anchor for pulling traction*

Knee Fractures

Fractures around the knee should be splinted from the hip to the ankle with a cylinder splint. You can use a life jacket or rolled-up sleeping pad, or foam from a berth or cushion. Individuals with fractures near the knee should not be allowed to walk without crutches.

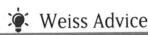 **Weiss Advice**

Knee and Lower Leg Immobilizer

Wrap an Ensolite pad or other type of sleeping pad around the lower leg from the knee to the foot. Fold the pad so that the top of the leg is not included in the splint. This allows for better visualization of the extremity and leaves room for swelling (**Fig. 48**).

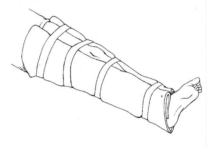

Fig. 48 *Knee and leg immobilizer*

Lower Leg (Tibia and Fibula) Fractures

As with other suspected fractures, examine for crepitus (grinding sounds), point tenderness, and immediate swelling.

Signs and Symptoms

A person with a tibia fracture will not be able to bear weight. Some people with an isolated fibula fracture can still walk on the injured leg but with pain.

Treatment

If necessary, apply gentle traction to straighten any deformity that exists in the leg and maintain the traction while another person applies a splint. For lower-leg fractures, apply a splint that includes the knee and ankle. An excellent splint is a U-shaped splint, with adequate padding, running from the inner thigh above the knee around the bottom of the foot and up the outside of the leg to above the other side of the knee. After splinting, elevate the leg to reduce swelling. Check the circulation and sensation in the foot every 30 minutes.

Ankle and Foot Fractures
It can be hard to differentiate a broken ankle from a severe ligament sprain without X-rays. Both injuries can produce swelling, pain, and black-and-blue discoloration.

Signs and Symptoms
If the person is unable to bear weight on the injured foot without significant pain, or if gentle pressure directly on the bony prominences ("bony bumps") on the inside or outside of the ankle produces severe pain, treat the injury as a fracture.

Treatment
Apply a well-padded splint that begins halfway down the calf and extends around the bottom of the foot and back up the other side, encompassing the ankle like a sandwich. The ankle should be splinted at 90 degrees (**Fig. 49**). Leave the boot or shoe in place, but remove the tongue so that circulation and sensation can be checked periodically. Keep the foot elevated above the level of the heart as much as possible.

Fig. 49
U-shaped splint for immobilizing a broken ankle or one of the bones in the lower leg

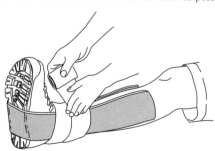

Toe Fractures
Signs and Symptoms
A fractured toe is swollen and usually becomes black-and-blue from underlying bleeding and most often is deformed compared to the adjacent toes. It is painful to move or bear weight on it.

Treatment
Splint a fractured toe by buddy-taping it to the adjacent larger toe with pieces of tape. Place cotton or gauze material between the toes to prevent rubbing and chafing. Toe fractures and dislocations are the most common injury aboard sailboats and motorboats. Wear protective footwear all the time, especially when walking on slippery decks, in rough seas, or on deck at night.

DISLOCATIONS
A dislocation is a disruption of a joint in which a bone is pulled out of its socket. Dislocations often damage the supporting structures of the joint and tear ligaments. Sometimes a bone under strain may pop out of position in the joint and back in again (subluxation). This will be painful but does not require reduction (relocation or returning of the bones to normal position). A subluxation is treated as a sprain injury. Dislocations are most common in the shoulders, elbows, fingers, and kneecaps (patella).

There are many good reasons for reducing a dislocation in the wilderness, or when voyaging in remote locations or offshore:

- Reduction is easier soon after injury, before swelling and muscle spasm develop.
- Reduction relieves pain.
- Early reduction reduces the risk of further injury to blood vessels, nerves, and muscles. Blood vessels can become trapped, stretched, or even compressed during a dislocation, which leads to loss of blood flow to the limb if reduction is not performed.
- It is easier to splint the extremity and evacuate the person after reduction.
- It is a technique one can learn to do with proficiency.

Even if a fracture accompanies the dislocation, the first step in treatment is to attempt to reduce the dislocation (although a fracture may sometimes prevent reducing the dislocation).

If you are unable to reduce the dislocation immediately, administer pain relievers and muscle relaxers; wait at least 20 minutes for the drugs to take effect, and for the person to perhaps recover from the initial shock of the injury, then try again. Use steady, constant traction when attempting a reduction, and tell the injured individual what you are going to do so the person will be better able to relax physically and mentally and work with you. After reduction, splint the extremity in the same manner as for a fracture. If a dislocation can't be reduced, splint the extremity in the most comfortable position for the person.

Shoulder Dislocation

Shoulder dislocations are common in kayakers and skiers because paddles and ski poles place added force on the shoulder joint. For a shoulder dislocation to occur, the arm is usually pulled away from the body, rotated outward, and extended backward. This can occur when a kayaker braces high or attempts to roll the boat. The arm gets yanked out of its socket and lodges in front of the joint.

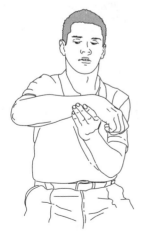

Signs and Symptoms

People with shoulder dislocations are usually in severe pain and aware that something is out of joint. The shoulder may look squared off, lacking the normal rounded contour. The injured person will usually hold the arm away from the body with the uninjured arm and be unable to bring it in tightly into

Fig. 50 *The victim with a dislocated shoulder holds the arm up and away from the body and is unable to bring the arm in against the chest, as one would for splinting.*

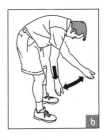

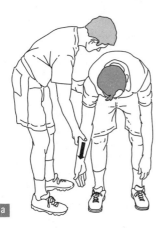

Fig. 51
One-person Weiss technique (standing) for reducing a dislocated shoulder

the chest (**Fig. 50**). If the person can bring the arm and hand across the body in a normal position for splinting and touch the opposite shoulder with that hand, then you should assume a shoulder dislocation is not the problem.

Treatment

Before attempting to reduce the shoulder, check the pulse in the wrist (radial pulse) and the circulation (temperature, color) in the hand. Check the nerve function by asking the person to move the wrist up and down and move all of the fingers. Test for sensation to touch or pinprick.

Many good techniques are used to reduce shoulder dislocations. The key is to do it quickly, before the muscles spasm.

Weiss Technique for Shoulder Reduction (Standing)

1. Have the person bend forward at the waist, while you support the chest, and allow the arm to hang down toward the ground. Support as much of the person's weight as possible to allow the person to relax.
2. With your other hand, grab the person's wrist and turn the arm slowly so that the palm faces forward. Then apply steady downward traction and very slowly bring the arm forward toward the head (**Fig. 51**). Avoid jerky movements. You may need to hold

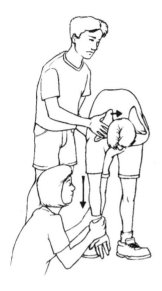

traction for a few minutes before it pops back into the shoulder socket.

3. If two medics are available, one should support the person at the chest and provide counter-traction while the other pulls downward on the arm. The person supporting the chest can also use the thumb of the other hand to push the scapula (shoulder blade) inward toward the backbone (**Fig. 52**). This scapular manipulation maneuver helps position the socket so the arm can slip back in easier.

4. You will usually notice a clunk and shift of the arm as it returns to the joint, combined with a sigh of relief from the person.

Fig. 52 *Two-person Weiss technique (standing) for reducing a dislocated shoulder*

One-Person Shoulder Reduction (Sitting)

1. While the person is sitting, grab the forearm close to the elbow with both of your hands.
2. With the person's elbow bent at 90 degrees, create traction on the arm by pulling steadily downward on the forearm.
3. After about a minute of sustained traction, slowly raise the entire arm upward, until reduction is complete.
4. Gingerly rotating the forearm outward while pulling in traction may facilitate reduction.
5. If available, another medic should provide counter-traction from behind the person while performing scapular manipulation as described in the preceding steps (**Fig. 53**).

After the shoulder is reduced, recheck the person's circulation, sensation, and ability to move the fingers and wrist. Immobilize the arm with a sling-and-swath bandage. After a shoulder dislocation is reduced, and the person needs to use the arm to facilitate exit from the wilderness (such as a kayaker needing to paddle to a take-out), a shoulder support can be used to help protect the injured shoulder (see "Shoulder SPICA," page 74).

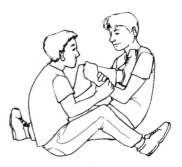

Fig. 53 *One-rescuer Weiss technique (sitting) for reducing a dislocated shoulder*

WARNING: If a dislocated shoulder cannot be reduced after two attempts, or if the reduction maneuver produces a dramatic increase in pain, the attempt should be aborted and the arm splinted in the most comfortable position for the person. This usually requires placing a pillow or rolled blanket under the armpit, between the arm and chest wall.

Elbow Dislocation

Signs and Symptoms

There is deformity of the elbow when compared with the uninjured side, and movement of the elbow is limited and painful. Check for a pulse in the wrist and determine if the person can move the fingers and wrist.

Treatment

Elbow dislocations require a great deal of traction and may be impossible to reduce in the wilderness. If you are unable to reduce the dislocation, splint the arm in the most comfortable position for the person. To attempt reduction, have the person lie on the stomach with the elbow bent at 90 degrees over the padded edge of a table or ledge. Pull downward on the wrist while another medic pulls upward on the upper arm (**Fig. 54**, page 116). Rocking the forearm back and forth gently may

help the reduction. After any
reduction attempt, recheck the
pulse in the wrist and circulation
to the fingers.

After reduction, the elbow
should be splinted as though it
were a fracture (see page 98).

Finger Dislocation
Signs and Symptoms
Someone with a dislocated
finger will be unable to move the
dislocated joint and a deformity
will be obvious. Do not attempt
to reduce a dislocation at the
base of the index finger. Splint
this injury in a position of comfort and seek medical attention.

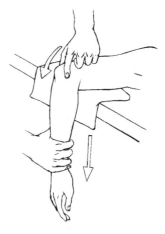

Fig. 54 *Reducing a dislocated elbow*

Treatment
Pull on the tip of the finger with one hand, while pushing the base
of the dislocated finger with the other hand (**Fig. 55**). After reduction,
buddy-tape the reduced finger to an adjacent finger (**Fig. 37**, page 100).

Note: Do not attempt to reduce a dislocation at the base of the
index finger. Splint this injury in a position of comfort and seek medical
attention.

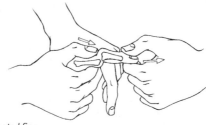

Fig. 55
Reducing a dislocated finger

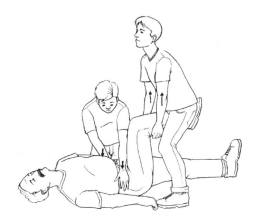

Fig. 56   *Reducing a dislocated hip*

Hip Dislocation

Signs and Symptoms

In most hip dislocations, the femur is pushed out and back, dislodging behind the pelvic socket. The person's leg is rotated inward, appears shortened, and the hip and knee are both flexed. The person experiences severe pain and is unable to move or straighten the injured leg.

Treatment

Two people and a lot of force are required to reduce a hip dislocation. Treat the person with pain medication and muscle relaxants. Place the person faceup with the knee and hip both flexed at 90 degrees. One medic will hold the person flat on the ground, or deck, by pushing down with the hands on both sides of the person's pelvic bone. The other medic straddles the person's calf, locks the hands behind the person's knee, and applies steady traction in an upward direction (**Fig. 56**). Reducing a hip is often difficult and requires a great deal of prolonged pulling to overcome the powerful leg muscles.

Once reduced, the injured leg should be splinted to the uninjured leg and the person transported to a medical facility. If reduction is unsuccessful, splint the leg in the most comfortable position for the person, then arrange evacuation.

Kneecap (Patella) Dislocation

Dislocation of the kneecap usually occurs from a twisting injury while the knee is extended.

Signs and Symptoms

The kneecap is displaced to the outer part of the knee, resulting in an obvious deformity and pain. The knee is usually flexed, and the person is unable to move it.

Treatment

A patella dislocation can usually be reduced by pushing the kneecap back toward the inside of the knee with your thumbs, while gently straightening the leg (**Fig. 57**). The kneecap will pop back into place, and relief from pain should be immediate. If the maneuver is very painful or not easily accomplished, do not continue. After the kneecap is repositioned, the person should be able to walk with an improvised knee immobilizer. If you're unable to reduce the patella, splint the knee in a position of comfort and evacuate the person.

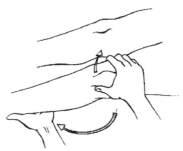

Fig. 57 *Reducing a dislocated kneecap*

Knee Dislocation

Do not confuse this devastating injury with a dislocation of the kneecap (patella).

Signs and Symptoms

A total knee dislocation disrupts all of the ligaments of the knee and results in a very unstable joint.

Treatment

Often the knee will reduce itself spontaneously. If the knee is still deformed, gently reposition and straighten it by applying gentle traction to the lower leg. Immobilize the joint with a splint applied to the back of the knee from mid-thigh to the calf, then evacuate the person as soon as possible.

Note: A major artery in the leg is often torn or damaged during the dislocation, and if not repaired within 6 to 8 hours, the leg may require amputation.

Ankle Dislocation

Signs and Symptoms

Sometimes a severe ankle fracture can also be dislocated. The foot or ankle looks twisted, bent out of shape, or out of its normal position. It is painful to bear any weight; an X-ray will be required to fully define the extent of the injury.

Treatment

Apply gentle traction to the foot and ankle until the deformity has been corrected and the ankle is better aligned. Splint the ankle as you would for a fracture.

WOUNDS: CUTS, ABRASIONS, AND BLISTERS

Managing Wounds

There are six goals to managing wounds in the backcountry or at sea:

- Stop bleeding
- Prevent infection
- Promote healing

- Permit continued function
- Reduce discomfort
- Verify that tetanus immunization is up to date (booster every 7 to 10 years)

Controlling Bleeding

Applying direct pressure to the wound can stop almost all bleeding. Use whatever clean material is available to hold pressure on the bleeding site. Then, as time allows, use sterile gauze from your medical kit. The idea is not to soak up blood with a big wad of bandage but, rather, to apply firm pressure directly on the bleeding site. If direct pressure does not stop the bleeding, examine the wound to make sure you are holding pressure on the correct spot before putting more bandages on top of those already in place. It might be necessary to hold pressure for up to 30 minutes to prevent further bleeding. If you need to free up your hands, create a pressure dressing by wrapping an elastic wrap bandage tightly around a stack of 10 x 10-cm (4 x 4-inch) gauze pads placed over the wound.

If bleeding from an extremity cannot be stopped by direct pressure, and the person is in danger of bleeding to death, apply a tourniquet. A tourniquet is any band applied around an arm or leg so tightly that all blood flow beyond the band is cut off. While a person is in the water, using a tourniquet may be necessary; applying direct pressure is almost impossible, especially while bringing a person to a boat or to shore, such as after a shark attack. Tying a surfboard leash or dive mask strap around a massively bleeding limb can be lifesaving. If the tourniquet is left on for more than 4 hours, everything beyond the tourniquet will likely die, and that part of the arm or leg may require amputation (see "How to Apply a Tourniquet," page 22).

Never apply direct pressure to a bleeding neck wound, because it can interfere with breathing. Instead, carefully pinch the wound closed. Never apply direct pressure to the eye, because you could cause permanent damage.

Anytime you deal with blood, it's vitally important to wear barrier gloves to protect yourself from blood-borne pathogens, such as hepatitis and HIV. Even latex gloves can leak, so make sure to wash your hands or wipe them with an antimicrobial towelette after removing the gloves. Dispose of bloody gloves and bandage materials by securing them in a waterproof bag.

When bleeding cannot be controlled with direct pressure, a QuikClot Sport hemostatic agent and QuikClot Emergency Dressings are useful products to apply to a bleeding wound. QuikClot Sport, an over-the-counter product, contains zeolite, a naturally occurring mineral that has been preloaded with moisture to eliminate the heat buildup that was present in the first generation of QuikClot products. QuikClot Sport's zeolite beads are contained in an easy-to-apply mesh pouch to be placed directly into the bleeding wound. QuikClot's third-generation products, available by prescription only, contain kaolin, a naturally occurring, inert mineral; they are available in gauze dressings. When either zeolite or kaolin comes into contact with blood in and around a wound, it assimilates the smaller water molecules found in the blood, and activates and promotes blood clotting. With either product, once the dressing or mesh pouch is applied, direct pressure must still be maintained for it to be effective.

Celox granules are another product that can help stop bleeding. When poured into a wound, the granules mix with blood and form a gel-like clot. To apply Celox, pour the granules from a sterilized, sealed packet into the wound, then hold them in place with a gauze dressing. Apply a compression bandage by wrapping an elastic wrap bandage over the gauze and around the bleeding site.

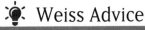

☀ Weiss Advice

Stopping the Bleeding

Oxymetazoline nasal spray (Afrin) contains a medication that constricts (shrinks) blood vessels and may help stop wound bleeding. Simply moisten a 10 x 10-cm (4 x 4-inch) piece of gauze with the solution, and then pack the gauze into the wound. A moistened, non-herbal tea bag may also help to control bleeding in the mouth; the tannic acid in tea acts as a blood-vessel constrictor and can even help relieve pain.

Cleaning Wounds

The moment skin is broken, bacteria begin to enter and multiply inside the wound, and any blood or damaged tissue left behind will create a feeding ground for hungry germs. The goal of wound cleansing, therefore, is to rid the wound of as much bacteria, dirt, and damaged tissue as possible. Because seawater is a rich broth of infectious microorganisms, polluting chemicals, plants, organic debris, and countless particles of synthetic materials, it should never be used to clean an open wound. Rivers, lakes, and ponds are similarly polluted to a varying degree. Therefore, treat all wounds that occur while engaging in water sports, even minor nicks, cuts, and scrapes, as contaminated and potentially serious; they require prompt and careful cleansing to prevent severe infections. Superficial minor scrapes, cuts, and abrasions should be cleaned with benzalkonium chloride (BZK) or similar antiseptic pads. Soap and water will also work for minor injuries.

The best cleansing method for a deeper wound is to attach an 18- or 19-gauge catheter tip to the end of a 20- to 35-mL syringe to create a high-pressure irrigation stream (see "How to Irrigate a Wound," page 123). Using the syringe like a squirt gun creates an ideal pressure, forceful enough to flush out germs and debris without harming tissues.

Disinfected water is ideal for irrigating wounds. Water can be quickly disinfected by adding 10 mL of 10% povidone-iodine (Betadine) solution to 0.5 L (1 pint) of fresh water and allowing it to sit for 5 minutes. If the water is particularly dirty, pour it through a coffee filter, bandanna, or paper towel before disinfecting it. Fresh tap water from the boat's water tank, unless it has been treated and passed through a galley filter, is neither sterile nor free of impurities. Disinfect it with 10% povidone-iodine (and filter if necessary) as described. Water stored in tanks filled by a reverse-osmosis desalinator is fine if the tanks and hoses are known to be clean. If in doubt, use a dilute povidone-iodine solution. An alternative to using the ship's water is to store 4 L (1 gallon) of commercial bottled water specifically for wound irrigation. Eyewash solution is another alternative. It is sterile, nonirritating, and excellent for irrigating wounds.

Hydrogen peroxide, alcohol, and Mercurochrome should not be poured into wounds, because they damage tissue and can delay healing (although dilute hydrogen peroxide's effervescent effect can be useful to clean coral cuts). Hydrogen peroxide's effect is degraded by light, temperatures above 29°C (85°F), and agitation. Even 10% povidone-iodine used full strength is toxic to delicate skin tissues and should not be poured directly into a wound unless diluted first.

How to Irrigate a Wound

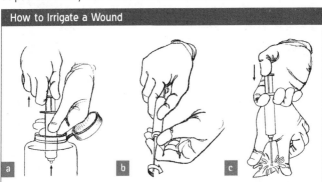

Fig. 58 *Wound irrigation*

Draw disinfected water into a syringe and attach an 18-gauge catheter tip. Hold the syringe so the catheter tip is just above the wound and perpendicular to the skin surface. Push down forcefully on the plunger while prying open the edges of the wound with your gloved fingers, then squirt the solution into the wound. Be careful to avoid getting splashed by the solution as it hits the skin (put on sunglasses or goggles to help protect your eyes from the spray). Repeat this procedure (**Fig. 58**) until you have irrigated the wound with at least 0.5 L (1 pint) of solution. Dirtier wounds require more irrigation. The more you use the better.

For wounds acquired in the marine setting and other contaminated wounds, after irrigation, gently spread the edges of the wound open and vigorously scrub the interior of the wound using a gauze pad soaked in clean disinfected water, cut away any dead or crushed tissue, then irrigate again. Inspect the irrigated wound for any residual particles of dirt or dried blood and, if present, carefully pick them out with tweezers. These steps will remove organic and inorganic debris and are crucial, because even one or two particles of dirt left in a wound will increase the likelihood of infection. Any renewed bleeding should again be controlled by direct pressure.

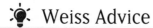 Weiss Advice

Wound Irrigation with a Plastic Bag and Safety Pin

Fill a plastic sandwich or garbage bag with disinfected water and puncture the bottom of the bag with a safety pin or pointy knife. Hold the bag just above the wound and squeeze the top firmly to begin irrigating.

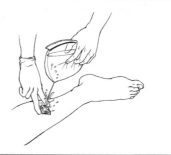

Closing Wounds

Many cuts can be closed safely in the backcountry or at sea. Time is a critical factor, however, and the longer you delay closure, the more likely the wound is to become infected after it is closed. The "golden period" for closing most wounds is within 8 hours after the injury occurs. If you wait longer, bacteria may enter and multiply inside the wound and interfere with the body's healing and defense system. Wounds on the face or scalp can be closed up to 24 hours later, because these areas are more resistant to infection. Many wounds are best left open—they will close themselves over time if kept clean and dressed with a barrier bandage.

Closing minor soft-tissue wounds is desirable to reduce the risk of infection and achieve a better cosmetic result; however, wound closure is never necessary. Infections that develop in closed wounds usually are considerably worse than those in open wounds. Never close a wound with sutures or staples if it was acquired in ocean water or contaminated (soaked) with seawater. If you elect to close it, use wound closure strips (see "Closing a Wound with Wound Closure Strips," page 126), and do not close the wound tightly.

Some wounds always carry a high risk of infection, regardless of when they are closed, and therefore they should be left open. Examples are wounds inflicted by animals, including marine creatures (e.g., sharks, eels, fish), human bites, puncture wounds, deep wounds on the hands or feet, and those that contain a great deal of crushed or damaged tissue. Wounds containing embedded foreign material (e.g., coral debris, sand, sea urchin spines, or fragments of clothing) should also be left open to drain. Any soft tissue wound that penetrates beyond the yellow layer of fat is likely to involve the fascia, the tough shiny white layer, and the tissue beneath it (muscle, tendon, bone, or joint). If you see white or red tissue in the wound, it is a deep wound and should never be closed because of the high risk of infection by entrapped bacteria. If in doubt about the risk of infection, do not close a wound.

High-risk wounds, and those that have aged beyond the 8-hour golden period, are best left open and packed daily (or more frequently, as needed) with 10 x 10-cm (4 x 4-inch) gauze dressings moistened with saline solution or disinfected water. (Seawater is not the same as physiological saline. A saline solution can be made by adding 9 g [1½ teaspoons] of table salt to 1 L [1 quart] of disinfected water.) Cover the packed wound with a bandage and splint the extremity. Consider puncture wounds high-risk, because they are difficult to clean. Begin hot soaks in fresh clean water for 15 minutes four times daily. The water temperature should not cause discomfort; aim for about 40.5°C (105°F). Antibiotics, if available, should be taken for all high-risk wounds. Begin cephalexin (Keflex) 500 mg four times daily for 5 to 7 days. Always seek medical consultation when treating high-risk wounds.

The preferred way to close a cut is with wound closure strips or butterfly bandages. Wound closure strips are better, because they are stronger, longer, stickier, and more porous than butterfly bandages.

Closing a Wound with Wound Closure Strips

1. Do not shave hair right next to the wound edge, as it abrades the skin and increases the potential for infection. Use scissors to clip hair near the wound so the tape will adhere better. Shave hair farther from the wound edge.

2. Apply a thin layer of tincture of benzoin or other topical skin adhesive, such as rosin, evenly along both sides of the wound, being careful to avoid getting the solution into the wound (it stings). Benzoin's stickiness will help keep the tape in place (**Fig. 59a**).

3. After the benzoin dries (about 30 seconds), remove a wound closure strip from its backing (**Fig. 59b**) and place it on one side of the wound. Use the other end of the strip as a handle to pull the wound closed (**Fig. 59c**). Try not to squeeze the wound edges tightly together; they should just touch. Attach the other end of the strip to the skin to keep the wound closed.

4. Overlap the wound edge with the wound closure strip by about 2.5 cm (1 inch) on each side. More strips can be applied as needed, with a gap of about 1 cm (0.5 inch) between each strip (**Fig. 59d**).

5. Place additional wound closure strips or pieces of tape crossways (perpendicular to the other strips) over the ends of the existing strips to keep the ends of the strips from curling up (**Fig. 59e**).

6. Leave the strips in place 7 to 10 days.

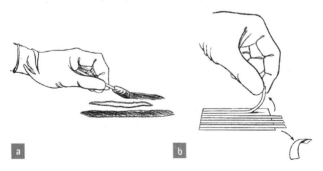

Fig. 59 *Applying wound closure strips*

☀ Weiss Advice

Improvised Wound Closure Strips

Wound closure strips can be improvised from duct tape, sail repair tape, or other adhesive tape. **1.** Cut 0.5-cm (0.25-inch) strips, then puncture tiny holes along the length of the tape with a safety pin to prevent fluid from building up under the tape. **2.** If you do not have tape, you can use superglue to attach strips of cloth or nylon from your clothes to the skin. Place a drop of glue on the material and hold it on the skin until it dries. **3.** Use the other end to pull the wound closed and glue it onto the skin on the other side of the wound. Avoid getting any glue in the wound. The glue is generally safe on intact skin but should not be used on the face. Expect the strip to fall off after about 2 to 3 days. You can reapply more strips with fresh glue if you are still traveling.

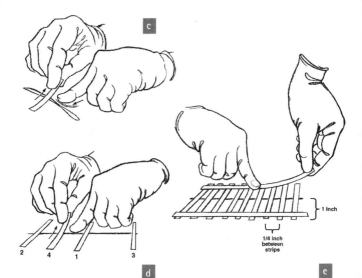

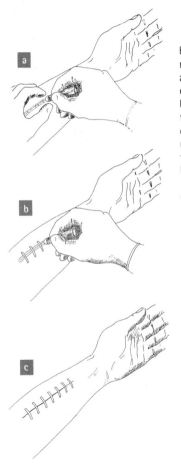

Using Tissue Glue (Dermabond) to Close a Wound

2-octyl cyanoacrylate (Dermabond) is a topical skin adhesive to repair skin lacerations. It is packaged as a small single-use applicator. Dermabond is ideal for use because it precludes the need for topical anesthesia, is easy to use, doesn't require needles, and takes up a lot less room than a conventional suture kit. It is expensive, but it can be purchased without prescription in single-dose vials. Over-the-counter (OTC) tissue glues (Nexcare Liquid Bandage Drops) can also be used, but they are not as strong an adhesive as Dermabond, and the wound edges are less likely to stay shut. OTC glues are suitable for small cuts (less than 2.5 cm [1 inch]) that are not under tension, where the edges come together naturally. When applied to the skin surface, Dermabond will keep wound edges stuck together for 3 to 4 days, and peels off without leaving evidence of its presence. Do not substitute a superglue for Dermabond, because that may cause injury to the skin (see **Fig. 60**).

1. Irrigate the wound with copious amounts of disinfected water.

Fig. 60 *Using glue and wound closure strips to close a wound*

2. Control any bleeding with direct pressure (the glue will not hold well when it is applied to a bleeding wound).

3. Apply tissue glue only to the outside surface of the wound to bridge over the edges; do not apply it directly into an open wound.

4. Gently squeeze the two wound edges together with your fingers so that they are straight, just touching each other, and lying together evenly. Be sure that the wound edges are matched correctly. Hold gauze against downstream areas to catch any drips as you apply the glue (**Fig. 60a**).

5. While you hold the edges together, have an assistant paint the tissue glue over the opposed wound edges using a very light brushing motion of the applicator tip. Avoid excessive pressure of the applicator on the tissue, because this could separate the skin edges and allow glue into the wound.

6. Apply multiple thin layers (at least three), allowing the glue to dry about 2 minutes between each application.

7. If the wound is large and difficult to approximate with your fingers, you can first use wound closure strips (see "Closing a Wound with Wound Closure Strips," page 126) to close the wound edges, and then glue between the strips (**Fig. 60b**). Next, remove one strip at a time and glue the skin where the strip used to be.

8. Glue can be removed from unwanted surfaces with acetone or loosened from skin with petrolatum jelly. (Do not use petroleum-based ointments and salves, including antibiotic ointments, on the wound after gluing, since these substances can weaken the glue and cause the wound to reopen.)

9. After the wound has been glued shut, apply or reapply wound closure strips to back up your closure (**Fig. 60c**).

10. Glue can be reapplied every few days over previous layers if necessary.

Large gaping cuts, and wounds that are under tension or that cross a joint are difficult to tape or glue closed and may require suturing or stapling. It helps to splint the joint or injured area to promote healing and maintain the integrity of the wound closure. Consult a physician for guidance regarding these options.

Using Staples to Close a Wound

Scalp, trunk, and extremity lacerations can also be closed with surgical skin staples. This method is versatile, inexpensive, and worth learning for anyone planning a trip to a remote area or an extended ocean voyage. Staples work as well as sutures, and sometimes better. Stapling is an excellent way to rapidly close a superficial (not deep) linear laceration (a clean, sharply defined cut). The wound should be properly cleaned and irrigated (see "How to Irrigate a Wound," page 123). Standard anesthetic agents should be used if available to make this process more comfortable, but they are not required. A topical lidocaine pad can be used as a substitute to swab the cut.

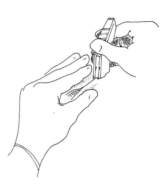

Fig. 61 *Applying gentle downward pressure to staple a wound closed*

The following steps are used to insert staples (**Fig. 61**):

1. Forceps or a gloved (sterile) hand is used to bring together the wound edges, which should be turned slightly outward (everted) and not tucked into the wound. An assistant can be very helpful in doing this while the primary operator uses the stapler.
2. The stapler should be placed on the skin over the wound, perpendicular to the surface.
3. Apply gentle downward pressure; avoid pushing down too hard and indenting the skin (**Fig. 61**).
4. The trigger (handle) should be gently and evenly squeezed to insert the staple into the tissue.
5. To release the device from the staple, relax thumb pressure fully and lift the stapler away from the skin.
6. Place the staples about 0.5 cm (0.25 inch) apart.
7. Dress the wound as described in the next section.

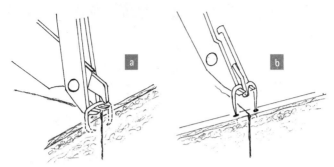

Fig. 62a *Slide jaws under staple*   **Fig. 62b** *Squeeze handle and lift*
and lift slightly.   *staple out.*

Staple removal (**Fig. 62**) requires a special disposable device (resembling a tiny pair of pliers). The lower jaws of the staple-removing device are positioned under the staple crossbar. Lift the staple slightly so that the staple is perpendicular to the surface (**Fig. 62a**). Continue slight lifting while gently squeezing the handles together to reform the staple. The upper jaw will compress (indent) the staple and open the loop. The staple can then be easily lifted up from the tissue and gently withdrawn (**Fig. 62b**). No anesthetic is required.

Inspect the stapled wound daily and change the dressing. If there are signs of infection, remove the staples and pack the wound with gauze dressings moistened with sterile saline or disinfected water. The recommended interval for removal of staples in adults is as follows:

- Scalp: 6 to 8 days
- Chest and abdomen: 8 to 10 days
- Back: 12 to 14 days
- Arm: 8 to 10 days
- Leg: 8 to 12 days

Note: Scalp lacerations can often be closed by stapling or by tying the person's hair together (see "Weiss Advice: Hair-Tying a Scalp Wound Closed," page 51).

Removing a Fishhook

Clean the site with dilute 10% povidone-iodine (Betadine) solution. Fishhooks with multiple hooks should have the free points taped or cut to avoid accidentally embedding them during removal. Anything attached to the hook (e.g., bait, line, lure) should be removed.

Pass a length of string, fishing line, suture material, or dental floss through and around the bend of the hook. Grasp the ends of the string and, while applying gentle downward pressure on the shank to disengage the barb, apply a firm, quick jerk of the string parallel to the shank (**Fig. 63a**). The fishhook may fly out, so wear eye protection and keep yourself and bystanders away from the hook's flight path. This maneuver can also be performed with Vise-Grip pliers instead of string.

If the string-yank technique fails, more invasive methods should be tried. Administration of a local anesthetic or application of ice over the area where the fishhook has penetrated may provide comfort, but neither is necessary for performing the procedure. The needle-cover technique is most effective for superficially embedded large hooks with a single barb (**Fig. 63b**). Advance an 18-gauge (or larger) needle along the track of the fishhook (parallel to the part of the shank ending with the barb); the bevel of the needle should face the barb. When the bevel of the needle covers the point, the barb is disengaged. The fishhook and needle are then removed at the same time.

The most successful technique (and sometimes the most painful) for large hooks, especially when the point is located near the surface of the skin, is the advance-and-cut technique. One could even make a shallow incision over the point under the skin to allow easier

Fishhook Injuries

Fishhooks are curved and have a barb just behind the tip, so the more force is applied to the hook, the deeper it penetrates. The barb does not allow the hook to be backed out. The classic method of advancing the barb through the skin and cutting the hook so that the remaining shank can be backed out is effective, but there is an easier and less painful technique (see "Removing a Fishhook," above).

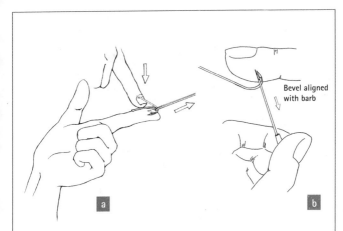

Fig. 63 *Removing a fishhook with the string technique*

penetration. Using pliers, the point and barb are advanced through the skin, and the point removed with cutters (use eye protection). The remaining shank is then backed out. After removing the hook, clean the entry point with an antiseptic towelette or soap and water. Monitor the puncture wound for signs of infection.

CAUTION: Fishhooks embedded in the eye should be left in place and secured with tape, the eye covered with a metal patch or cup, and the person transported to an ophthalmologist for definitive care.

Dressing Wounds

The best initial dressing is one that won't stick to the wound. Many nonadherent dressings are available over-the-counter.

Allowing the wound to dry out and form a scab delays healing. A slightly moist (not wet) environment is preferable to a dry one. Apply an antibiotic ointment to reduce infection and promote healing: bacitracin zinc and polymixin B sulfate (Polysporin) or mupirocen (Bactroban)

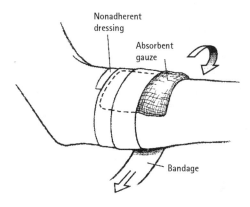

Fig. 64 *Dressing and bandaging a wound*

to cuts and abrasions and silver sulfadiazine (Silvadene) to burns. Then apply a nonadherent dressing to the wound, and place an absorbent gauze dressing over the nonadherent one. Hold these both in place with a conforming roller bandage, such as Coban (**Fig. 64**). Change a dressing whenever it becomes wet or dirty. If the wound is subject to movement, especially if on a hand, on a foot, or over a joint, immobilize it with a splint to promote healing.

Water sports enthusiasts need durable, waterproof dressings to keep a wound dry. When practical, wear dishwashing gloves over hand wounds and lightweight water-repellent gear over the injured areas. The objective is to keep saltwater and fresh water out of the wound. Small injuries, including blisters, small cuts, and nicks that are not deep, and abrasions, can be covered with New-Skin. This waterproof liquid antiseptic bandage has both pain-reducing and antibacterial properties. Apply the liquid in multiple layers. It will remain intact for several days. Tegaderm is a breathable, transparent, and waterproof dressing ideally suited for covering wounds in the aquatic environment. Whenever possible, use waterproof adhesive tape. One of the best waterproof tapes for the marine environment is plastic-coated cloth tape made by Johnson & Johnson.

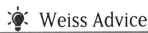

Weiss Advice

Making a Nonadherent Dressing

A nonadherent dressing can be made by spreading an antibiotic ointment over one side of a 10 x 10-cm (4 x 4-inch) gauze dressing. Honey can also be used in place of the antibiotic ointment. When applied topically, it can reduce infection and promote wound healing.

A conforming roller bandage can be improvised from a shirt or other article of clothing by cutting a thin strip of material in a circular fashion.

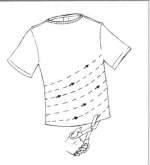

Cut a T-shirt in a circular fashion.

Check Wounds Daily for Signs of Infection

Even wounds closed under ideal circumstances have about a 5 percent chance of becoming infected. Wounds that are frequently wet have an even greater likelihood of infection, so check daily for the following signs of infection:

- Increasing pain, redness, or swelling
- Pus or greenish fluid drainage from the wound
- Red streaks on the skin adjacent to or "upstream" from the wound
- Fever

If signs of infection develop, remove the tape or staples, and open the wound to allow drainage. Pack the wound with moist gauze daily and begin cephalexin (Keflex) 500 mg four times a day. Medical consultation is advisable if there is no response to the antibiotic in 24 hours and the infection appears to be spreading.

Abrasions (Road Rash)

An abrasion occurs when the outer layer of skin is scraped off. Abrasions are often embedded with dirt, sand, bits of coral, and other debris, which, if not removed, can result in scarring or infection.

An abrasion must be vigorously scrubbed with a surgical brush or cleansing pad until all foreign materials are removed. This can sometimes be more painful than the accident itself. It helps to first spread a topical anesthetic, such as 4% lidocaine (Xylocaine) jelly, over the

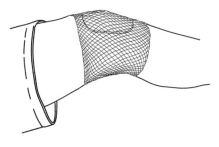

Fig. 65 *Stockinette bandage*

wound or wipe the area with a cleansing pad containing lidocaine. Use tweezers to pick out any remaining embedded particles, then irrigate the abrasion with saline solution or water. A thin layer of aloe vera gel applied to the abrasion after cleaning will reduce inflammation and promote healing.

After cleansing, apply a nonadherent, protective dressing and secure it in place with a bandage. GlacierGel Blister & Burn Dressings or Spenco 2nd Skin work well, because they soothe and cool the wound while providing an ideal healing environment. GlacierGel dressings feature a 50% hydrogel dressing pad with an adhesive film layer attached for easy application. You can secure Spenco 2nd Skin with a stockinette or nonwoven adhesive knit bandage (**Fig. 65**). Either dressing can be left in place for several days, as long as there is no sign of infection.

Splinters

Splinters are a common injury among boaters while working on wood boats and using wood docks. These wounds become easily infected when neglected or when splinters are removed with dirty instruments, such as a pocketknife.

Prevention

To prevent these injuries, wear protective gloves while working with wood. Be sure tetanus immunization is up to date; a booster of adult tetanus and diphtheria (Td) vaccine is required every 7 to 10 years to maintain immunity.

Treatment

If the splinter protrudes above the surface, remove it with forceps or tweezers, swab the skin with an antiseptic pad, and treat the injury as a puncture wound. Splinters just under and parallel to the skin surface can be teased out with the sharp beveled edge of an 18- or 20-gauge needle after cleansing the skin with antiseptic. After removal, treat according to the instructions for wound management (see "Managing Wounds," page 119). Deeper splinters require medical consultation for surgical exploration and removal. Observe the puncture site and treat early infection (see "Staph and Strep Infections: Cellulitis," page 145).

To remove a splinter that lodges entirely under the fingernail with no part protruding, try the following technique: Insert the tip of a sterile 23- or 25-gauge needle directly into the end of the splinter, bevel side up, with the needle roughly parallel to the nail plane. Next, lower the hub (the plastic) of the needle; this should bring the needle tip toward the nail edge and drag the splinter along with it. Completing this motion should bring the splinter out along with the needle.

Blisters

Prevention

Eliminate as many contributing factors as possible:

- Make sure that shoes and deck boots fit properly. A shoe or boot that is too tight causes pressure sores; one that is too loose leads to friction blisters.
- Break in new boots and deck shoes gradually before your trip.
- Wear a thin liner sock under a heavier one for extended hiking. Friction will occur between the socks instead of between the boot and the foot. If you're out of dry sock liners, use a plastic sandwich bag as a friction-reducing layer (allow it to remain folded on itself). Always wear socks when wearing deck boots.
- Avoid prolonged wetness, which breaks down the skin, predisposing it to blisters. Dry feet regularly and apply a moisturizing lotion to hands and feet.

- Before hiking or boating, apply moleskin or Molefoam to sensitive areas where blisters commonly occur.
- When you begin paddling, wear paddling gloves until your hands toughen.
- Wear sailing gloves to handle lines until hands toughen.

Treatment of Small, Intact Blisters

1. If the blister is small and still intact, do not puncture or drain it.
2. Place a piece of moleskin or Molefoam, with a hole cut out of the middle and slightly larger than the blister, for placement over the blister. The material should be thick enough to keep the shoe from rubbing against the blister. This may require several layers. Secure this with tape.

Treatment of Large or Ruptured Blisters

1. If the bubble is intact, puncture it with a clean needle or safety pin at its base and massage out the fluid. The fluid contains inflammatory juices that can delay healing.
2. With scissors, trim away any loose skin from the bubble.
3. Clean the area with an antiseptic towelette or soap and water.
4. Apply antibiotic ointment or aloe vera gel, and cover with a non-adherent dressing or a gauze pad. Spenco 2nd Skin, GlacierGel Blister & Burn Dressings, and Compeed hydrocolloid dressings are all excellent, commercial blister dressings.
5. Place a piece of Molefoam, with a hole cut out slightly larger than the blister, around the site. Secure everything with tape or a piece of nonwoven adhesive knit dressing. Change the dressing daily or every other day. First applying a topical adhesive (benzoin or rosin) to the skin around the blister will help hold the Molefoam in place.
6. Inspect the wound daily for any sign of infection. This includes redness around the wound, swelling, increased pain, or cloudy fluid collecting under the dressing. If this occurs, remove the dressing to allow drainage. Begin cephalexin (Keflex) 500 mg four times a day. Consult a physician if there is no response to the antibiotic in 24 hours and the infection appears to be spreading.

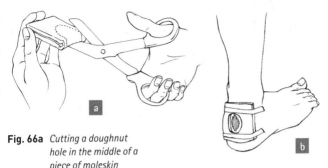

Fig. 66a *Cutting a doughnut hole in the middle of a piece of moleskin*

Fig. 66b *Covering a hot spot or blister with moleskin*

Hot Spots

Hot spots are sore, red areas of irritation which, if allowed to progress, develop into blisters.

1. Take a rectangular piece of moleskin (soft cotton flannel with adhesive on the back) or Molefoam (which is thicker and somewhat more protective than moleskin), and cut an oval-shaped hole in the middle (like a doughnut) the size of the hot spot (**Fig. 66a**).
2. Center this over the hot spot and secure it in place, making sure that the sticky surface is not on irritated skin. This will act as a buffer against further rubbing (**Fig. 66b**).
3. Reinforce the moleskin with tape or a piece of nonwoven adhesive knit dressing.

☀ Weiss Advice

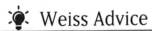

Moleskin and Molefoam Substitute Before Hot Spots

If moleskin or Molefoam is not available, place a piece of tape over the hot spot (duct tape works well). Molefoam can be even be improvised from a piece of padding, while a piece of material from the cuff of a sweatshirt or flannel shirt can be used as moleskin.

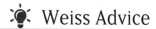

Weiss Advice

Gluing a Blister Back in Place

If you are far from help, must continue walking, and only have a tube of superglue or benzoin, consider this option: Drain the fluid from the blister with a pin or knife and inject a small amount of glue or benzoin into the space that you have evacuated. Press the loose skin overlying the blister back in place and cover the site with tape or a suitable dressing. The extreme pain this produces will only last a few minutes.

BURNS

The severity of the injury is related to the size and depth of the burn and the part of the body that is burned. First-aid treatment and the necessity for evacuation are based on the overall burn size in proportion to the person's total body surface area (TBSA).

The Rule of Nines or the Rule of Palms (**Fig. 67**) can estimate the size of the burn injury.

Rule of Nines (Adults)

- Each upper extremity = 9 percent of TBSA
- Each lower extremity = 18 percent of TBSA
- Front and back of trunk each = 18 percent of TBSA
- Head and neck = 9 percent TBSA
- Groin = 1 percent

Rule of Palms

An individual's palm covers an area roughly equivalent to 1 percent of the body surface area. Use the size of the person's palm as a measure to estimate the percentage of body area burned.

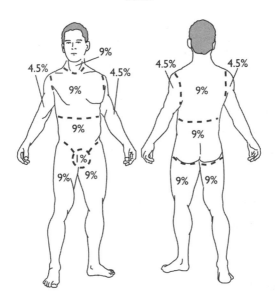

Fig. 67 *Rule of Nines body divisions*

General Treatment
1. Apply cool fresh water to the area. Do not overcool the person and produce hypothermia. Do not use ice except on very small burns.
2. Assess the airway and do primary and secondary surveys.
3. Remove all burned clothing from the person.
4. Remove any jewelry from burned hands or feet.
5. For chemical burns, flush the site with large amounts of water for at least 15 minutes.
6. A person with a burn greater than 20 percent TBSA can lose a great deal of fluids from burned tissues and can go into shock. Encourage the person, if not vomiting and consciousness is normal, to drink fluids.

7. Burns less than 5 percent TBSA (excluding second-degree burns of the face, hands, feet, or genitals, or those completely encircling an extremity) can be treated in the wilderness or at sea if adequate first-aid supplies are available and wound care is performed diligently.

First-Degree Burns (Superficial Burns)
Signs and Symptoms
Only the outermost layer of skin is involved. There is redness of the skin and pain, but no blisters are present. Sunburn is an example, as are most spilled-coffee burns and rope burns.

Treatment
1. Cool the burn with wet compresses (do not use ice directly).
2. Apply aloe vera gel topically to the burn.
3. Anti-inflammatory drugs (ibuprofen [Advil, Motrin] 600 mg three times a day [with food] for 3 days) will provide pain relief and speed healing.
4. First-degree burns rarely require evacuation.

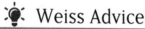

☀ Weiss Advice

Covering Burns with Honey

A gauze pad covered with honey is an effective covering for burns. It reduces infection and promotes healing of the wound.

Second-Degree Burns (Partial-Thickness Burns)
Signs and Symptoms
This is a deeper burn, resulting in both redness and blistering. Blisters may not occur for several hours following injury. The burned area is quite painful and sensitive to touch.

Treatment
1. Irrigate the burn gently with cool water to remove all loose dirt and skin.

2. Peel off or trim with scissors any loose skin.
3. Large—greater than 2.5-cm (1-inch)—thin, fluid-filled blisters should be swabbed with an antiseptic pad and drained with a sterile needle, and the dead skin trimmed away. Small, thick blisters may be left intact.
4. Apply aloe vera gel or silver sulfadiazine (Silvadene) antibiotic cream to the burn.
5. Cover the burn with a nonadherent dressing, such as Spenco 2nd Skin, Telfa, or Xeroform. Change the dressing at least once a day.

GlacierGel Blister & Burn Dressings are 50% water–based gel dressings on a waterproof and breathable adhesive film. They are easy to apply and last up to 4 days. GlacierGel dressings eliminate pain from blisters and burns, and the clear gel dressing allows you to monitor the blister or burn site for infection.

Third-Degree Burns (Full-Thickness Burns)
Third-degree burns involve all layers of the skin, including nerves, blood vessels, and even muscle.

Signs and Symptoms
Although these are the most serious burns, they are not painful, because the nerve endings have been destroyed. The skin next to a third-degree burn may have suffered only a second-degree burn and still be painful. The appearance is usually dry, leathery, firm, and charred when compared with normal skin, and insensitive to light touch or a pinprick. Third-degree burns require skin grafting.

Treatment
1. Treat as for second-degree burns.
2. Watch for shock if the burn is extensive.
3. Evacuate the person.

Prevention of Burns Aboard Sailboats and Motorboats
- The leading causes of fires on boats are AC and DC wiring faults. The most common electrical problem is related to chafed wires.

Battery cables, bilge pump wires, and even instrument wires chafing on hard objects, such as vibrating engines or sharp-edged bulkheads, start many fires. AC heaters and other household appliances that have been brought onboard cause a small number of fires every year. Overheated engines start a quarter of boat fires. Review the electrical and engine systems at regular intervals for maintenance and safety.

- Skin burns commonly occur from accidentally touching or brushing against exposed hot engine components.

Prevention of Burns While Cooking in the Galley on a Moving Boat

- Do not cook in rough weather.
- Use heavy pots; pressure cookers are ideal.
- Use a gimbaled stove, and secure the cookware to the stovetop.
- Secure covers on pots and pans to prevent splashing of hot food and liquids.
- Wear a protective rubber apron and shoes or boots.
- Place hot dishes on a nonskid surface.
- Transfer hot liquids in a deep sink.
- Keep a fire blanket and fire extinguisher in the galley.
- Avoid using alcohol stoves, because they flare up.

Prevention of Burns While Handling Lines under Tension

- Avoid friction burns by keeping a couple of turns on the winch while raising, lowering, and trimming sails.
- Maintain tension on the bow cleat or anchor windlass when paying out the anchor line.
- Wear sailing gloves to handle ropes until hands toughen, or in wet, rough conditions.

SKIN PROBLEMS

Skin infections occur in hikers, divers, paddlers, and sailors where areas of skin break down due to friction, pressure, and trauma. Once started, these infections can spread to other people via direct contact with infected skin or other contaminated surfaces (e.g., clothing, towels, wet suits, and dive equipment).

Prevention
- Use antibacterial soaps when bathing, and dry off thoroughly.
- Avoid sitting around in a wet bathing suit.
- Change moist socks and underwear frequently.
- Wear clothing that wicks away moisture and breathes.
- Use emollients (Lubriderm or Neutrogena cream) to prevent skin cracking and areas of friction.
- Treat all skin injuries, even minor ones, as possibly contaminated, and carefully follow the principles and procedures for wound care on land and in the marine environment.

Staph and Strep Infections: Cellulitis

Streptococcus (strep) or *Staphylococcus* (staph) bacteria are the most common cause of wound infections both on land and in the marine environment. They are normally found in saltwater and fresh water and on human skin. Bacteria enter the deeper layers of the skin through scratches, cuts, and abrasions that are not carefully cleaned and treated. Infection often starts in minor cuts and injuries on the hands and feet. Bacteria in the wound multiply and reach sufficient numbers to overwhelm the body's defenses.

Signs and Symptoms

Signs of spreading cellulitis (subcutaneous infection of connective tissue) are expanding areas of redness (usually with well-defined borders), swelling, warmth, and tenderness. Pus is often present in the wound. Red streaks in the skin may appear, leading from the wound up the arm or leg toward the heart. Lymph nodes draining the area (usually in the armpit or groin) become enlarged and tender. Untreated, bacteria can enter the bloodstream and spread throughout the body, producing life-threatening infections in the internal organs. At this stage the person experiences high fever, shaking chills, lethargy, and loss of appetite; headache, nausea, vomiting, and diarrhea may also be present. A simple skin infection can quickly progress to a medical emergency, requiring evacuation and hospitalization.

Treatment

1. Open and thoroughly clean any wound; if it was closed with wound closure strips, sutures, or staples, remove them.

2. Scrub the wound vigorously with soap and water or dilute povidone-iodine (Betadine) solution daily, and allow drainage by packing it with absorbent gauze covered by a dry dressing.

3. Apply warm compresses for 20 minutes four times a day to the surrounding affected area, and elevate the arm or leg to promote circulation and drainage.

4. Maintain hydration, and minimize activity with the affected extremity.

5. Immediately begin oral antibiotics: cephalexin (Keflex) 500 mg four times daily or amoxicillin clavulanate (Augmentin) 875 mg twice daily. Treat for 7 to 10 days until the infection has completely cleared. Azithromycin (Zithromax) is also effective; take two 250 mg tablets on day 1, then 1 tablet daily for 5 days; restart on day 8 if the infection is not completely resolved.

6. Outline the infected skin area with a ballpoint pen or marker to visualize the response to oral antibiotics. The affected red and tender area should begin to recede, and the swelling and pain should diminish. If spreading continues after 24 to 36 hours of treatment, evacuation will be necessary, however, consider adding sulfamethoxazole combined with trimethoprim (Bactrim DS), one tablet twice daily to treat drug-resistant bacteria.

7. If blisters develop—especially if they appear blood filled or darken to blue, purple, or black—a marine bacterial infection may be present (see "*Vibrio vulnificus* Infections," page 148). Add ciprofloxacin (Cipro) 750 mg twice daily or levofloxacin (Levaquin) 500 mg daily and seek medical consultation.

Staph and Strep Infections: Impetigo
Signs and Symptoms
Impetigo begins as a red bump, progresses to a blister, and develops into a localized, crusted yellow lesion.

Treatment
1. Systemic antibiotics include cephalexin (Keflex) 500 mg four times daily; amoxicillin clavulanate (Augmentin) 875 mg twice daily; and 2 azithromycin (Zithromax) 250 mg tablets on day 1, then 1 tablet daily for 4 days; restart on day 8 if the infection is not completely resolved. Alternatively, mupirocin (Bactroban) cream can be applied to small lesions.
2. The lesions are highly contagious, so cover the area with a dressing until healed.

Staph and Strep Infections: Folliculitis and Boils
Signs and Symptoms
Infections start in the hair root and appear as a pimple. They may swell with pus to form an abscess (boil), which may require incision and drainage in addition to oral antibiotics. These lesions most commonly affect the neck, breasts, buttocks, groin, armpits, and waist.

Treatment
1. Small pimples are best treated early with topical mupirocin (Bactroban) cream.
2. Use systemic antibiotics for multiple, extensive, and deeper infections: cephalexin (Keflex) 500 mg four times daily; amoxicillin clavulanate (Augmentin) 875 mg twice daily; or 2 azithromycin (Zithromax) 250 mg tablets on day 1, then 1 tablet daily for 4 days; restart on day 8 if the infection is not completely resolved.
3. A soft abscess contains pus. Apply warm soaks to bring it closer to the surface—a white or yellow area where the pus may be visible under the skin—and encourage it to drain spontaneously.
4. If the infected site remains painful and fails to drain, clean the overlying skin with full-strength 10% povidone-iodine (Betadine)

and nick the top with a sterile scalpel blade or beveled needle. Gently express the pus (using a nonsterile glove is okay) and irrigate the abscess cavity with sterile water. Do not try forcefully squeezing the abscess to pop it, as you may drive the infection into the deeper tissues.

5. Continue soaks and antibiotics and cover with a sterile dressing to absorb any additional pus and fluid. The infection will quickly resolve after drainage.

Vibrio Vulnificus Infections

The *Vibrio vulnificus* bacteria thrives in saltwater or brackish warm water. It is found in all U.S. and worldwide coastal waters. *Vibrio vulnificus* causes the most potentially lethal infection of all marine bacteria.

Signs and Symptoms

The infection often begins with a puncture wound or cut made by a fish, crab, oyster, or barnacle. Skin lesions begin as painful, rapidly advancing swollen red areas, which develop blisters, pus, and ulceration. The distinctive blood-filled blisters turn into open draining blue-black sores, with dead skin at the center. High fever is usually present. Untreated, the bacteria can enter the bloodstream and large areas of adjacent tissue. This may be fatal in people especially susceptible to this organism (e.g., alcoholics, people on prolonged steroid medication or chemotherapy, and people with AIDS, cancer, leukemia, chronic liver disease, diabetes, or impaired immune systems).

Treatment

1. Immediately start ciprofloxacin (Cipro) 750 mg twice daily, or levofloxacin (Levaquin) 500 mg daily, for 7 to 10 days. Follow the guidelines for treatment of cellulitis.

2. Levofloxacin (Levaquin) is also effective against strep or staph, which makes it the ideal single drug for persons infected with *Vibrio vulnificus*. Consult a physician if you suspect this infection.

3. Hospitalization, with intensive antibiotic therapy and surgical drainage with excision of dead tissue, is often required.

Pseudomonas Infections: Hot Tub Folliculitis

"Hot tub folliculitis" is a skin infection associated with contaminated hot tubs, whirlpools, swimming pools, and spas.

Signs and Symptoms

The skin infection may be localized or widespread. Signs of infection include a diffuse, itchy, pus-filled, bumpy eruption on red, swollen patches of skin. It is most evident on areas covered with bathing suits, but it can occur anywhere. Rarely, a low-grade fever, sore throat, and headaches accompany the rash.

Treatment

This condition is self-limited and heals without specific therapy if one discontinues water-related activities and permits the skin to dry out.

Erysipelothrix (Fish-Handler's Disease)

A scratch, abrasion, or puncture wound acquired while handling fish (including shellfish) is a common source of this bacterial infection. The organism thrives in freshwater and saltwater.

Signs and Symptoms

The fingers and hands are commonly infected. The infection may spread down the finger, into the webbed space between the fingers, and up the next finger. It is rare to have the palm of the hand affected. Fever and swelling lymph nodes in the armpit of the affected arm are often present. The distinctive appearance is usually a painful, warm, itchy, swollen, red-to-violet circular area at the site of the puncture wound. Around this area, a clear area appears in a circle, surrounded by another raised, purplish, swollen area. If untreated, the infection may blister and spread to involve the entire hand, wrist, or forearm, causing cellulitis with swelling, redness, and pain.

Treatment

Treat as for cellulitis and begin antibiotics. Choices include cephalexin (Keflex) 500 mg four times daily, ciprofloxacin (Cipro) 500 mg twice daily, amoxicillin clavulanate (Augmentin) 875 mg twice daily, or levofloxacin (Levaquin) 500 mg daily. Treat for 7 to 10 days.

Mycobacterium Marinum Infections

This tuberculosis-like bacterium thrives in both freshwater and saltwater, irrigation ditches, aquariums, and swimming pools (it is not killed by chlorine). It often shows up weeks after the initial wound (cut, scrape, or puncture) and causes slow wound healing.

Signs and Symptoms

Fingers and toes are the most common sites of infection. The lesion can have several appearances. Often it presents as a raised red bump 1 to 2.5 cm (0.5 to 1 inch) wide, which becomes hard and scaly. The bump may open and drain. It can also appear as a line of bumps running up the affected limb. Diagnosis is difficult to make without a skin biopsy and culture.

Treatment

Treatment is required for 1 to 3 months depending on the severity: 2 azithromycin (Zithromax) 250 mg tablets on day 1, then 1 tablet daily for 4 more days; ciprofloxacin (Cipro) 500 mg twice daily; or doxycycline (Vibramycin) 100 mg twice daily are effective; however, it is best to consult with an infectious disease specialist before initiating treatment.

Fungal Infections: Jock Itch, Athlete's Foot, and Candidiasis

Prevention

Antifungal powders help to prevent infections. Keep skin areas prone to infection dry, and change socks and underwear frequently when moist. Avoid wearing a wet bathing suit for prolonged periods whenever possible.

Signs and Symptoms

The affected areas are moist red, itchy, and subject to secondary bacterial infection. Jock itch occurs in the groin, and athlete's foot occurs in the webbed area between the toes. Women may develop fungal infections under the breasts and in the vagina.

Treatment
1. For athlete's foot, terbinafine (Lamisil) or clotrimazole (Gyne-Lotrimin/Lotrimin) cream should be liberally applied to dry skin areas.
2. For vaginal infection, treat with fluconazole (Diflucan) 150 mg capsule (one dose) or miconazole (Monistat) cream and wear dry, breathable underwear.
3. For infection under the breasts, treat with nystatin (Mycostatin) cream or powder.

Fungal Infections: Tinea Versicolor (Pityriasis Versicolor)

Signs and Symptoms
Tinea versicolor (pityriasis versicolor), another skin fungus that thrives in heat and humidity, creates light-colored spots (called sun spots) as the surrounding area tans. It commonly grows on the neck, shoulders, chest, and back.

Treatment
Treat the areas with selenium sulfide (Selsun Blue) or ketoconazole (Nizoral) shampoo. To apply, wet the skin with water and rub the shampoo onto the affected area; let it dry for 10 minutes, wash it off, and reapply as directed.

Poison Ivy, Poison Oak, and Poison Sumac

Contact with poison ivy, poison oak, or poison sumac can cause an extremely itchy rash. The risk of developing a rash after exposure to these plants increases with each exposure. One's degree of sensitivity can change drastically from one exposure to the next. An individual may have no reaction or a minor rash one time, and then be incapacitated by a major breakout the next.

The offending resin is present in the plants year-round, even when they are only sticks or vines without leaves during the winter. The resin (oil) is also carried in smoke and can irritate the skin, mouth, eyes, and ears; it causes serious lung problems if inhaled. Boaters may be more vulnerable to the rash, because the protective barrier of natural skin oils is often washed away during aquatic activities. In general, poison

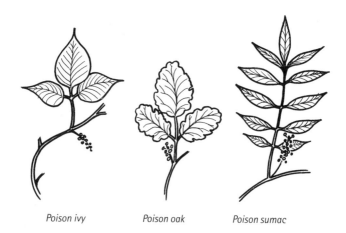

Poison ivy   *Poison oak*   *Poison sumac*

ivy grows east of the Rockies, poison oak grows west, and poison sumac grows best in the southeastern United States. The plants do not grow in Alaska and Hawaii, nor do they survive well above 1200 m (4000 feet), in deserts, or in rain forests.

The leaflets on poison ivy and poison oak grow in clusters of three leading to the saying, "Leaflets three, let them be." Poison oak has three to five leaflets, and poison sumac has seven to thirteen. All species have a cluster of green fruit in the angle between the leaf and twig of origin. Poison ivy leaves are initially bright green; they turn yellow and then bright red in the fall. Oak leaves vary from green to red.

Both poison ivy and poison oak grow as small or tall shrubs or vines. The poison ivy vine can wind around a tree trunk or stretch across the ground. Poison oak is a low-growing shrub or woody vine. Poison sumac resembles a large shrub or small tree with leaflets turning red in the fall.

IvyBlock, an over-the-counter barrier cream that prevents the resin from touching the skin and also inactivates it, can provide some protection if placed on the skin at least 15 minutes before possible exposure to the plant, and then every 4 hours. The cream is of no use if the skin has already been exposed. Do not use this product on children younger than 6 years unless directed to do so by a physician.

The plant's sticky resin can stay active on clothing or shoes for many months, so contaminated clothing should be handled carefully and laundered immediately. In addition to clothing, resin adheres to paddles and gear that comes into contact with plants. Oil may float along the shoreline where leaves and roots trail from the bank into the water.

The resin binds to skin within minutes. It is best to wash it off immediately, and certainly within 10 to 15 minutes. After an hour it cannot be washed off with soap and water. Gentle washing with a solvent such as rubbing alcohol neutralizes the oil and may leach some out of the skin. Alcohol hand-sanitizing lotions (Purell) may be used, but do not use prepackaged alcohol wipes, as the amount of alcohol is insufficient. Washing with copious amounts of tepid water and plain soap will dilute the oil and render it harmless. Some solvents, such as Zanfel Poison Ivy Wash or Tecnu Oak-n-Ivy Outdoor Skin Cleanser, may remove the oil from the skin, even when used more than an hour after exposure, but they are expensive and may not always do the job.

Signs and Symptoms

The rash may take from a few hours to days to develop and starts as red, itchy bumps, followed by blisters that may become crusted. It can be streaky or patchy, and it "itches like crazy." It appears first where the concentration of resin was strongest and emerges over time on other areas of the body where it was less concentrated. This leads to the misconception that the oozing fluid from blisters or the skin spreads the rash. Scratching after you have washed the original oil from the skin cannot spread the rash. Scratching is still discouraged, because it can produce a secondary skin infection and also increase itching.

Treatment

1. If left untreated, the rash will clear in about 2 weeks.
2. Over-the-counter steroid creams (hydrocortisone cream) and calamine lotion may be useful for small patches of the rash but are ineffective for severe extended rashes. Prescription-strength cortisone cream is useful for treating small affected skin areas to prevent blister formation and ease the itching, but it should not be applied to the face or deep skin folds—use lower potency topical cortisone ointment in these areas.

3. Cool, wet compresses made with Domeboro Astringent Solution will provide some relief from the itching. Apply the soaks for 15 minutes four times daily, before using cortisone cream.

4. Oral antihistamines (diphenhydramine [Benadryl] 25 to 50 mg) every 4 to 6 hours will help relieve some of the itching, but will also cause drowsiness. Topical antihistamines (calamine lotion) will help as well.

5. For a widespread rash, or one involving the face or genitals, strong oral corticosteroid drugs such as prednisone (Deltasone and others) or a methylprednisolone pack (Medrol Dosepak) can be used. It takes about 12 hours for the drug to work, but once it does, the relief is dramatic. Side effects from a 2-week course of prednisone are generally mild and worth the benefit. One recommended dose schedule is to start 60 mg for 3 days, 40 mg for 3 days, 20 mg for 3 days, and complete with 10 mg for 3 days.

☀ Weiss Advice

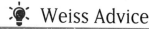

Removing Poison Ivy or Poison Oak from the Skin

Any solvent may help remove the oil of poison ivy or poison oak from the skin. Gasoline, paint thinner, and rubbing alcohol have all been reported to be effective; however, these products can themselves be irritating to the skin.

HEAD PROBLEMS
Headache

Headache is a common reason for seeking medical care. Headaches originate from innumerable causes, including tension and stress, migraine, excessive sun exposure, dehydration (see "Dehydration Headache," page 157), heat illness, altitude illness, alcohol hangover, carbon monoxide poisoning (see "Carbon Monoxide Hazards," page 238), brain tumors, strokes, aneurysms, intracranial bleeds, fever, flu, meningitis and other infectious diseases, high blood pressure, sinus infections (see "Sinus Infection (Sinusitis)," page 158), and dental problems (see "Dental Injuries and Emergencies," page 60). Suddenly going cold turkey on caffeine or alcohol during an offshore passage, especially if you regularly drink more than 3 cups of coffee a day or have multiple cocktails daily, can also precipitate a headache (see "Alcohol Withdrawal," page 186).

Tension Headache

This is the most common type of headache and affects people of all ages. Pain is related to continuous contractions of the muscles of the head and neck, and can last from 30 minutes to a week.

Signs and Symptoms

The headache is described as tight or viselike, felt on both sides and the back of the head and neck. The pain is not made worse by walking, climbing, or performing physical activity. Sensitivity to light may occur, but fever, nausea, and vomiting are not present.

Treatment

Loosen any tight-fitting hats. Ibuprofen (Advil, Motrin) 600 mg or acetaminophen (Tylenol) 1000 mg every 4 to 6 hours may help relieve the discomfort. A neck and scalp massage may be beneficial together with heat packs to the back of the neck. For a sustained tension headache, try lorazepam (Ativan) 0.5 to 1 mg every 6 hours to reduce muscle tension and anxiety.

Migraine Headache

The term *migraine* is often used as a catchall phrase but should be reserved for those headaches that show specific patterns.

Signs and Symptoms

These recurrent headaches usually start during adolescence and typically involve only one side of the head, but not always, and are associated with nausea, vomiting, and sensitivity to light. Walking or physical exertion makes the pain worse. About 15 percent of people with migraine headaches experience an aura (flashing lights, distorted shapes and colors, blurred vision, or other visual apparitions) prior to the onset of the headache.

Treatment

Ibuprofen (Advil, Motrin) 800 mg along with caffeinated beverages, such as coffee, may help relieve symptoms, especially if taken early. Stronger prescription medications, such as acetaminophen (Tylenol) with codeine, acetaminophen with hydrocodone (Vicodin), sumatriptan (Imitrex), or eletriptan (Relpax), may be needed. Ondansetron (Zofran) 4 mg oral dissolving tablet will help treat the nausea and vomiting. Lying down in the shade with a cool compress on the forehead may be helpful.

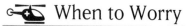 # When to Worry

Headaches

Some headaches may signal a life-threatening illness. Evacuate to a medical facility as soon as possible a person with any of the following symptoms:

- The headache is the worst ever, and came on suddenly and severely (aneurysms or intracranial bleeding).
- The arms and legs on one side are weak, numb, or paralyzed, or one side of the face appears droopy (stroke).
- It is impossible to talk or express oneself clearly (stroke).
- A fever, stiff neck, or rash is present (meningitis).
- The headache grows steadily worse over time (brain tumor or brain swelling from injury or bleeding).
- Vomiting is repetitive.
- Seizures or convulsions develop.
- The pain does not go away over a period of 24 hours.

Meningitis

This is a severe infection caused by a variety of organisms and involves the lining of the brain and spinal cord.

Signs and Symptoms

The headache of meningitis is severe and often accompanied by nausea, vomiting, fever, altered level of consciousness, and altered mental status, such as confusion and bizarre behavior. The neck is stiff and painful when the chin is flexed downward against the chest. An infant can suffer meningitis without a stiff neck and may manifest only poor feeding, fever, lethargy, and irritability.

Treatment
If meningitis is suspected, the person should be started on broad-spectrum antibiotics and evacuated. Oral antibiotics sometimes may be infective; however it is reasonable to start amoxicillin clavulanate (Augmentin) or ampicillin if available. This is a contagious and life-threatening illness that requires intravenous antibiotics.

Dehydration Headache
Headache can be an early sign of dehydration.

Signs and Symptoms
The pain is felt on both sides of the head and is usually made worse when the person stands from a lying position.

Treatment
Resting and drinking at least 1 to 2 L (1 to 2 quarts) of water should relieve the pain. On average, you need to drink about 1.5 to 2 L (1.5 to 2 quarts) a day, and more if perspiring in tropical climates or with increased activity in warm weather. Drink sports drinks, which contain salts and sugar to replace fluid losses. A good barometer of your hydration status is the color of your urine; if it is not clear or very light tan, then you're not drinking enough (see "Illnesses Caused by Heat," page 221).

Sinus Headache
Signs and Symptoms
Sinus headache is usually associated with a sinus infection and typified by fever, nasal congestion, production of nasal discharge, and pain in the front of the face. Tapping over the sinuses over the eyebrows or at the upper part of the cheek may increase the pain.

Treatment
See "Sinus Infection (Sinusitis)," page 158.

Sinus Infection (Sinusitis)

Infection of the sinuses may accompany a cold or hay fever.

Signs and Symptoms

The most prominent symptom is a frontal headache or feeling of heaviness above the eyes or adjacent to the nose. Drainage into the nose or back of the throat, nasal congestion, low-grade fever, and tenderness with pressing over the infected sinus are clues to a sinus infection. Pain may be felt in the upper jaw or teeth.

Treatment

Antibiotics, such as amoxicillin clavulanate (Augmentin) and azithromycin (Zithromax), are recommended. Use an oral decongestant (pseudoephedrine [Sudafed]) or nasal spray (oxymetazoline [Afrin]), and seek medical consultation if no improvement is made.

EYE PROBLEMS

Conjunctivitis

Conjunctivitis often results from a viral or bacterial infection on the inside of the eyelids and the whites of the eyes.

Signs and Symptoms

Chemicals found in swimming pools, sunscreens, soaps, and seawater, as well as particles in the eye, can also cause inflammation, which is difficult to distinguish from an infectious cause. Pinkeye, a highly contagious bacterial infection, makes one or both eyes red and itchy; a thick yellow-green discharge oozes from the eyes and during sleep can glue the eyelids shut. The lids become inflamed, swollen, and crusty.

Treatment

1. Isolate towels and washcloths, and wash hands after instilling eyedrops.
2. Instill two drops of ofloxacin (Floxin) into each eye four times a day for 5 days after irrigating the eye with eyewash or clean tap water.
3. Warm compresses over the closed eye are also soothing.

4. Remove contact lenses and wear sunglasses outdoors to protect the eyes from wind and dust.
5. If the red eye does not respond to therapy, or if a change in vision occurs, seek medical consultation.

Styes or Abscesses
Signs and Symptoms
Styes or abscesses on the eyelid produce localized swelling, redness, and pain.

Treatment
1. When a stye begins to develop, apply warm, moist compresses to the eyelid for 30 minutes four times a day, until the stye either disappears, or enlarges and comes to a head. If it comes to a head but does not drain spontaneously, seek medical attention.
2. If more than 48 hours from medical care and the infection is progressing to include the cheek or forehead, carefully lance the stye with a scalpel or sterile needle. This should be followed by antibiotic therapy; start cephalexin (Keflex) 500 mg four times daily, and continue warm soaks for 10 minutes four times daily.

THROAT PROBLEMS
Tonsillitis ("Strep Throat")
Signs and Symptoms
Signs and symptoms that suggest bacteria (rather than a virus) as the cause of a sore throat include high fevers (over 39°C [102°F]); a grayish-white coating on the tonsils or pus in the back of the throat; muffled voice; burning sensation in the throat; and enlarged lymph nodes in the front of the neck.

Treatment
Bacterial sore throats are treated with antibiotics such as cephalexin (Keflex), amoxicillin clavulanate (Augmentin), or azithromycin (Zithromax). Acetaminophen (Tylenol) and lozenges help to relieve throat pain. Adults can also dissolve 2 aspirin in warm water, and gargle for 3 minutes as needed.

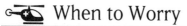 # When to Worry

Sore Throat

If the person cannot swallow saliva or open the mouth fully, evacuation as soon as possible to a medical facility for treatment is necessary. Antibiotics, if available, should be administered en route.

EAR PROBLEMS
Middle Ear Infection (Otitis Media)
Signs and Symptoms
Symptoms include throbbing or stabbing pain in the ear, decreased or muffled hearing, and fever. Occasionally, a yellow discharge may drain from the ear.

Treatment
Treatment consists of an oral antibiotic (such as amoxicillin clavulanate [Augmentin], azithromycin [Zithromax]) for 7 days, and a decongestant, such as pseudoephedrine (Sudafed). To reduce the pain and swelling, especially in children, fill the ear canal with benzocaine (Auralgan), then moisten a cotton plug with benzocaine and insert that into the opening of the canal; repeat as needed every 2 hours.

Swimmer's Ear (Otitis Externa)
Swimmer's ear is an infection of the outer ear canal caused by water and bacteria.

Prevention
To prevent swimmer's ear, maintain dry, slightly acidic (that's where vinegar helps) ear canals, and keep the skin intact. Dry the canals well with a soft towel after swimming, and pull on the earlobes while tilting the head to help water run out. If necessary, use eardrops (e.g., Swim-EAR) to evaporate water from each ear canal after swimming. A similar solution can be made by mixing equal parts of rubbing alcohol and vinegar or, equally effective, 2% boric acid and alcohol. Some people use a drop or two of mineral oil or lanolin in the canals to prevent the canal

from drying out. Avoid inserting a cotton swab to clean or dry the canal; it packs wax into the far end of the canal, further trapping moisture and bacteria, and damages the delicate skin of the inner ear canal. Earplugs irritate the canal in the same way. Earwax and earplugs can trap air in the canal in front of the eardrum and prevent equalization on descent or ascent, which can lead to a ruptured eardrum.

Signs and Symptoms

The first sign is usually itching and vague discomfort in the ear canal. Within a few hours to a day, the ear can become red and extremely painful and drain yellowish fluid. Pain is elicited if you pull down on the earlobe, push on the small flap of ear that covers the canal, or push against the outer ear. Sudden severe ear pain during or after a dive represents a ruptured eardrum, not swimmer's ear, and eardrops should not be used (see "Barotrauma: Injuries of Descent," page 248).

Treatment

Make an irrigating solution by mixing equal parts of rubbing alcohol and vinegar, then with gentle pressure, irrigate the ear canal using a syringe until it is clear of debris (the solution coming out of the ear will become clear).

If you don't have rubbing alcohol, try 1 part vinegar diluted with 4 parts clean water. Stand in a breeze and allow the ear to dry. Follow this by instilling a few drops of Domeboro Otic, a drug with antibacterial properties. If pain persists, use ofloxacin otic (Floxin) or another antibiotic eardrop, and repeat four times a day and at bedtime. Keep water out of the ear for 2 to 3 weeks or until the inflammation clears.

RESPIRATORY INFECTIONS

Bronchitis

Bronchitis is an infection of the air passages leading from the windpipe to the lungs. It is often caused by the same viruses that are responsible for colds.

Signs and Symptoms

The major symptom is a cough that may be dry or produce yellow or greenish phlegm. Pain in the upper chest, which worsens with coughing or deep breathing, is sometimes present. People with uncomplicated bronchitis usually are not short of breath and do not have a rapid respiratory rate.

Treatment

1. Cough expectorants that help bring up phlegm may be useful. Cough suppressants, such as codeine, that impair the body's normal process for expelling phlegm should be reserved for nighttime use to allow for better sleep.
2. Drink plenty of fluids to help thin the mucus and make it easier to expel.
3. Most cases of bronchitis are caused by viruses, which do not respond to treatment with antibiotics. Colored sputum (brown, yellow, green) often signifies a bacterial infection, and the antibiotics amoxicillin clavulanate (Augmentin), azithromycin (Zithromax), or cephalexin (Keflex) can shorten the duration of infection.

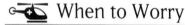 # When to Worry

> **Cough**
>
> If you develop shortness of breath, fever above 38ºC (101ºF), wheezing, severe pain in the chest, or a cough producing blood-specked or greenish phlegm, you should begin treatment for pneumonia and obtain medical consultation.

Pneumonia

Pneumonia is an infection of the lungs usually caused by either a bacteria or virus.

Signs and Symptoms

Symptoms include a cough that usually produces green or yellowish phlegm, fever, shaking chills, and weakness. Stabbing chest pain that is often made worse with each breath, shortness of breath, and rapid breathing may also occur.

Treatment

1. Children can be treated with amoxicillin 40 mg per kilogram (1 kg = 2.2 pounds) in three divided doses.
2. Levofloxacin (Levaquin) and azithromycin (Zithromax, Zithromycin) are the preferred drugs in adults, because they treat the broadest variety of organisms causing pneumonia.
3. Maintain hydration and administer expectorants as suggested for bronchitis; obtain medical consultation if the person has persistent high fevers, shortness of breath, difficulty breathing, or chest pain after 24 to 48 hours of treatment.
4. Certain pneumonias require specific antibiotics or combination of drugs.
5. Pneumonia can be a fatal illness in persons with reduced immunity, chronic lung disease, and other major illnesses. It is always recommended to seek medical advice when treating these persons.

SEIZURES

Seizures (convulsions) can result from drugs, tumors, head injury, heat illness, low blood sugar, fever in children, or other causes.

Signs and Symptoms

Normally, a grand mal (full body) seizure lasts 2 to 3 minutes, during which the person is unresponsive. When the seizure ends, the person will be sleepy and confused. Obtain medical consultation as soon as possible. Be sure persons with chronic seizure disorders have been taking their regular prescribed medications.

Treatment

1. Do not try to restrain convulsive movements.
2. Move harmful objects out of the way.
3. Make sure the airway is clear and the person is breathing. If not breathing, start mouth-to-mouth rescue breathing.
4. Roll the person into a side-lying position to protect the airway if vomiting occurs.
5. Do not put anything in the person's mouth.

INSULIN SHOCK AND DIABETIC KETOACIDOSIS

Diabetes is a disorder of carbohydrate metabolism usually characterized by inadequate production of the hormone insulin relative to the body's needs. The blood sugar is elevated, and excessive urine production, thirst, hunger, and weight loss follow. A diabetic who becomes confused, weak, or unconscious for no apparent reason may be suffering from insulin shock (low blood sugar) or diabetic ketoacidosis (high blood sugar).

Insulin Shock (Low Blood Sugar)

If a diabetic takes too much insulin or fails to eat enough food to match the insulin level or the level of exercise, a rapid drop in blood sugar can occur. Low blood sugar may also result from a mismatch of the dose of oral diabetic medications and food intake.

Signs and Symptoms

Onset of seasickness with loss of appetite, nausea, and vomiting makes blood sugar control difficult for a diabetic and predisposes to low blood sugar. Symptoms—ranging from weakness, slurred speech, bizarre behavior, and loss of coordination to seizures and unconsciousness—may come on very rapidly.

Treatment

If still conscious, the person should be given something containing sugar to drink or eat as rapidly as possible. This can be fruit juice, candy, or a nondiet soft drink. If the person is unconscious, place sugar granules, honey, or glucose paste from your first-aid kit under the tongue, where it will be rapidly absorbed.

Diabetic Ketoacidosis (High Blood Sugar)

Diabetic ketoacidosis (formerly called diabetic coma) comes on gradually and is the result of insufficient insulin. Usually the person has neglected to take a scheduled dose of insulin due to feeling ill and not eating. The stored sugar in the body is then released, and this eventually leads to a very high sugar level in the blood.

Signs and Symptoms

Early symptoms include frequent urination and thirst. Later, the person becomes dehydrated, confused, or comatose and develops nausea, vomiting, abdominal pain, rapid breathing, and fruity breath.

Treatment

This condition requires evacuation as soon as possible to a medical facility in order to restore metabolic balance. If not vomiting, and awake and alert, the diabetic should take small sips of water frequently. If you are unsure whether the person is suffering from insulin shock (low blood sugar) or ketoacidosis (high blood sugar), it is always safer to assume it is low blood sugar and administer sugar. The person may have a blood sugar meter you can use to determine the blood sugar level (normal is 90–125). The person's history also can help you sort out this dilemma.

GASTROINTESTINAL PROBLEMS (ABDOMINAL PAIN AND BELLYACHES)

Abdominal pain can be due to many causes, including constipation, gas, infection, inflammation, internal bleeding, ulcers, and obstruction or leaking of major blood vessels. Abdominal pain can sometimes also be caused by pneumonia, a heart attack, kidney stones (see "When to Worry: Back Pain," page 86), or pelvic problems. The diagnosis can be difficult, even with the best diagnostic testing and clinical experience. When possible, obtain medical consultation early, and keep a log of symptoms, vital signs, and physical findings.

When to Worry

Abdominal Pain

Seek medical help for any abdominal pain that lasts longer than 4 to 6 hours or is accompanied by frequent or projectile vomiting (vomit that seems to come out under pressure), signs of peritonitis (see "Peritonitis," page 169) or fever. Some common causes of abdominal pain that require urgent medical evaluation are appendicitis, ulcer, bowel obstruction, pelvic infections, and any pain during pregnancy.

Appendicitis

The appendix is located in the lower right side of the abdomen. Appendicitis occurs when the appendix becomes inflamed and swollen and fills with pus. Appendicitis can occur in persons of any age, but it is most common in young adults.

Signs and Symptoms

The affected person usually has a vague feeling of discomfort that often begins in the center of the upper abdomen and within a matter of hours moves to the lower right side. Pain is persistent and steady but may be worsened by movement, sneezing, or coughing. Loss of appetite, nausea, fever, and occasionally vomiting are typical. Pressing the belly on the right lower side increases the pain.

Treatment

1. Evacuate the person as soon as possible. If evacuation will take longer than 24 hours and the person is not vomiting, administer small sips of water (no food) at regular intervals (every 15 minutes).
2. Administer broad-spectrum antibiotics such as levofloxacin (Levaquin) 500 mg once a day together with metronidazole (Flagyl) 500 mg four times daily.

Diverticulitis

Many adults (usually over 40 years old) have diverticula, small pea-size pouches scattered throughout the lining of the large intestine. The pouches sometimes become inflamed (similar to appendicitis), which produces diverticulitis. Dehydration, constipation, and a diet restricted in the roughage gained from fruit, salad, other vegetables, and fiber predispose someone with diverticula to this illness; on an extended cruise or paddling trip this is often the diet.

Signs and Symptoms

Pain is commonly located in the lower left or lower center of the abdomen, and tenderness is found when pressing those areas. Often, fever and diarrhea, sometimes containing small amounts of visible blood, are present. This clinical picture resembles some forms of traveler's diarrhea (see "Traveler's Diarrhea," page 174), and a detailed dietary history may help distinguish between the two illnesses.

Treatment
The bowel should be allowed to rest, with only fluids consumed for the first few days. Start levofloxacin (Levaquin) 500 mg daily. Add metronidazole (Flagyl) 500 mg every 6 hours if no improvement is seen within the first 36 to 48 hours. Improvement can be monitored by a reduction in fever, diarrhea, pain, and tenderness. Treatment should be continued for 7 to 10 days, with gradual introduction of a normal diet.

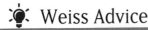

☀ Weiss Advice

Ulcer Pain or Heartburn

If you have ulcer pain or heartburn (acid indigestion) and are without any antacids, a glass of cold water alone will sometimes provide relief. A teaspoon or two of mentholated toothpaste, washed down, may provide some relief. Avoid toothpaste brands containing baking soda or hydrogen peroxide.

Stomach Ulcer
An ulcer is an erosion or crater that develops in the lining of the stomach or small intestine.

Signs and Symptoms
An ulcer usually produces persistent burning pain in the center of the upper abdomen. The pain is occasionally relieved by eating and is often associated with nausea, belching, and vomit that contains blood or looks like brown coffee grounds. Dark black stools may indicate that the ulcer is bleeding. Sometimes an ulcer can be painless. Similar signs and symptoms may occur with general inflammation of the lining of the stomach (gastritis) or of the esophagus.

Treatment

1. Administer acid-buffering medication, such as aluminum hydroxide–magnesium hydroxide (Maalox) and simethicone (Mylanta), or acid-reducing medication, such as cimetidine (Tagamet), famotidine (Pepcid), or ranitidine (Zantac). It is fine to use both for the first few days, especially if pain persists.
2. Avoid taking aspirin or anti-inflammatory drugs such as ibuprofen (Advil, Motrin).
3. Avoid alcohol, spicy foods, and tobacco.
4. Obtain medical consultation.

Bowel Obstruction

Bowel obstruction is a blockage of the intestines and occurs most commonly in individuals who previously have had abdominal surgery. It can also develop from infection as well as other causes.

Signs and Symptoms

Symptoms include nausea, vomiting, and cramping abdominal pain. The person's breath may have a fecal odor, and the abdomen may look and feel distended.

Treatment

Do not give the person anything to eat or drink. If evacuation is expected to take longer than 24 hours and the person is not vomiting, administer small sips of water at regular intervals (every 15 minutes) and administer antibiotics (levofloxacin [Levaquin] and metronidazole [Flagyl]).

Gallstones (Gallbladder Disease)

The gallbladder is connected to the underside of the liver in the upper right part of the abdomen, just below the ribs. Stones can form in the gallbladder and produce an obstruction to the flow of bile.

Signs and Symptoms

Pain and tenderness are present in the upper right side of the abdomen. Pushing under the rib cage on the right side of the abdomen while the person takes a deep breath will increase the pain. The pain may radiate to the shoulder or back. Nausea and vomiting usually occur. The pain may subside abruptly if the stone is passed.

Treatment
Although the condition is not immediately life-threatening, it is best to evacuate the person as soon as possible to a medical facility. Administer pain medication to the person and a broad-spectrum antibiotic, such as levofloxacin (Levaquin) 500 mg daily. Do not give the person anything to eat. If evacuation will take longer than 24 hours and the person is not vomiting, administer small sips of water at regular intervals (every 15 minutes).

Peritonitis
When an injured or diseased hollow organ begins to leak its contents (e.g., ruptured bowel, perforated stomach, burst appendix, inflamed gallbladder), peritonitis—a severe inflammation of the entire abdomen—develops.

Signs and Symptoms
The person quickly becomes extremely ill, with diffuse abdominal pain, tenderness, nausea, and vomiting, eventually going into shock. The abdominal muscles become very tense, making external examination difficult.

Treatment
With such an extreme emergency, one can do little but arrange evacuation as soon as possible. Do not give fluids, and administer the oral antibiotics levofloxacin (Levaquin) and metronidazole (Flagyl).

Vomiting
In the marine environment, vomiting is most often related to seasickness, but it also may be a sign of a more serious medical problem. If it persists, obtain medical consultation, especially in the presence of fever, abdominal pain, or abdominal tenderness.

Treatment

Drink small but frequent amounts of liquids, such as broth, juice, or diluted sports drinks. Avoid drinking too much too soon; that will cause the stomach to become distended, resulting in more vomiting. Avoid solid food until the vomiting has stopped. Use prochlorperazine (Compazine) 10 mg or promethazine (Phenergan) 25 mg suppositories every 6 hours if vomiting is recurrent or persists for more than an hour. Ondansetron (Zofran), an oral disintegrating tablet, is also very effective, acts quickly, and can be taken up to three times a day.

⚕ When to Worry

Vomiting

Obtain professional medical care immediately if vomiting is associated with any of the following:
- Head or abdominal trauma
- Severe lethargy or confusion
- Severe abdominal pain or distention
- Blood in the vomit or vomit with a coffee-ground appearance
- Fever higher than 38°C (101°F)
- Vomiting that continues for longer than 24 hours

Hemorrhoids

Hemorrhoids are enlarged veins found both outside and inside the anal opening.

Prevention

The best way to prevent hemorrhoids is to prevent constipation (see "Constipation," page 171).

Signs and Symptoms

Hemorrhoids can cause minor itching, severe pain, and bleeding.

Treatment

Hemorrhoids can be treated topically with specialized over-the-counter creams or suppositories. Any over-the-counter hydrocortisone cream will also be effective. Hemorrhoid pads with witch hazel are excellent for external hemorrhoids.

Constipation

Constipation (difficult bowel movements with hard stools) is a common problem when traveling in the wilderness or during extended ocean passages, due to disruption of normal habits.

Prevention

Constipation is easier to prevent than to treat. Drinking fluids to stay well-hydrated and adjusting the diet to include fruit, vegetables, and whole grains are helpful.

Treatment

If one is constipated, a stool softener can be used (e.g., mineral oil, psyllium), with or without a gentle laxative such as prune juice or magnesium hydroxide (milk of magnesia). When no stool has been passed for 5 to 10 days due to constipation, the stool may have to be removed from the rectum using a gloved finger, a suppository, or an enema. This should be done carefully to prevent injury to the anus and walls of the rectum.

Diarrhea

Diarrhea is an increase in the frequency and looseness of stools. Common causes of diarrhea include ingestion of food and water contaminated with viruses, bacteria, and parasites, such as *Giardia* and *Cryptosporidium*. Food sensitivities may arise without warning, and stress may also provoke diarrhea.

A major concern is the amount of fluid loss. The degree of dehydration can be estimated from certain signs and symptoms:

- *Mild dehydration (3 to 5 percent weight loss):* Headache, nausea, lethargy, light-headedness, thirst, dry mucous membranes (lips, mouth), normal pulse, and tan concentrated urine. This represents a 1 to 2 L (1 to 2 quart) deficit of body water in a 75-kg (165-pound) person.
- *Moderate dehydration (5 to 10 percent weight loss):* Thirst, dry mucous membranes, sunken eyes, small volume of dark urine, and rapid and weak pulse.

■ *Severe dehydration (greater than 10 percent weight loss):* Drowsiness or lethargy, very dry mucous membranes, sunken eyes, no urine, no tears, and shock (rapid pulse that is weak and difficult to feel) together with pallor and low blood pressure.

 # Weiss Advice

Rehydration Solutions

Try one of the following rehydration methods:

Rehydration Solution #1
Add 6 g (1 teaspoon) table salt, 12 g (4 teaspoons) cream of tartar (potassium bicarbonate), 2 g ($^1/_2$ teaspoon) baking soda, and 50 g (4 tablespoons) sugar to 1 L (1 quart) of drinking water.

Rehydration Solution #2
Alternate drinking two separate solutions, prepared in the following manner:
■ 250 mL (8 ounces) fruit juice, 2.5 mL ($^1/_2$ teaspoon) honey or corn syrup, and a pinch of salt
■ 250 mL (8 ounces) water and 1 g ($^1/_4$ teaspoon) baking soda

Treatment
1. *Replace fluids and electrolytes.* Oral rehydration, with water and oral rehydration salts (ORS), is the most important treatment for diarrhea illnesses. The fluids and electrolytes lost from the body with diarrhea can be potentially fatal in children and devastating in adults. The body can still absorb much of the water and electrolytes given orally, even during a severe bout of diarrhea. The fluid in diarrhea itself contains electrolytes, including sodium chloride (salt), potassium, and bicarbonate, so simply drinking plain water is inadequate replacement. Many sports drinks sold commercially are not ideal for replacement of diarrhea losses: the high concentration of sugar may increase fluid loss, and the electrolyte contents may not be optimal. Sports drinks can be used but should be diluted to half strength with water.

2. *The World Health Organization recommends oral rehydration solutions* that contain the following combination of electrolytes added to 1 L (1 quart) of water: sodium chloride 3.5 g; potassium chloride 1.5 g; glucose 20 g, and sodium bicarbonate 2.5 g.

3. *ORS packets* can be purchased commercially from medical kit suppliers and retail stores selling outdoor recreation supplies.

4. *Mildly or moderately dehydrated adults should drink* 4–6 L (1–1.5 gallons) of oral rehydration solutions in the first 4 to 6 hours. Children can be given 240 mL (1 cup) of ORS every hour. Severe dehydration usually requires evacuation to a medical facility and intravenous fluids.

5. *Rice, bananas, and potatoes* are good supplements to oral rehydration solutions. Fats, dairy products, caffeine, and alcohol should be avoided. Avoid drinking full-strength juices as a rehydration solution, since they usually contain three to five times the recommended concentration of sugar and can worsen the diarrhea.

6. *Antimotility drugs.* If the person does not have bloody diarrhea or a fever greater than 38°C (101°F), loperamide (Imodium) can be taken orally to reduce cramping and diarrhea. The dose for adults is 4 mg initially, followed by 2 mg after each loose bowel movement up to a maximum of 14 mg per day. Imodium is preferred over Lomotil, because it has fewer potential side effects. Imodium should not be given to children. Bismuth subsalicylate (Pepto-Bismol, Kaopectate) are other commonly used antimotility drugs that may be helpful.

7. *Antibiotics.* Antibiotics are recommended if diarrhea is accompanied by fever (38°C [101°F] or greater), if there is pus or blood in the stool, if the person has signs and symptoms of giardiasis (see "Giardiasis," page 176), or if the person is traveling in the developing world (see "Traveler's Diarrhea," page 174).

8. *Avoid contagion.* Don't spread the disease! Careful hand washing is a critical part of treatment to prevent possible reinfection, and infection of the crew and trip members. Everyone should use soap and water before eating and after every bowel movement; air-dry the hands. Avoid food preparation if ill, and do not handle group serving spoons and group food platters.

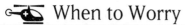 When to Worry

Diarrhea

Obtain medical assistance if diarrhea is accompanied by any of the following:

■ Blood or mucus in the stool
■ A fever greater than 38°C (101°F)
■ Severe abdominal pain or distention
■ Moderate to severe dehydration
■ Diarrhea lasting longer than 3 days

Traveler's Diarrhea

Traveler's diarrhea refers to diarrhea that occurs in the context of foreign travel. It usually occurs when people visit underdeveloped, or developing countries, and even "developed" European countries. *E. coli* is a common cause of this illness. Although most people make a full recovery, seven strains of *E. coli* identified around the world cause a potentially fatal illness in otherwise healthy people.

Prevention

Traveler's diarrhea, usually caused by bacteria, afflicts almost half of all visitors to underdeveloped countries. It is acquired through ingestion of contaminated food or water. Watching what you eat and drink may help but does not guarantee that you will not get sick.

■ Travelers should avoid drinking untreated tap water or drinks with ice cubes. Bottled and carbonated drinks are generally safe. Bottled noncarbonated water may be safe if the seal has not been broken, but exercise caution as unscrupulous street vendors have been known to sell bottled water that has not been disinfected.

■ Custards, salads, salsas, reheated food, milk, and peeled fruits and vegetables (when peeled and prepared by someone else) should be avoided. Diarrhea following certain foods suggests bacterial infection.

■ Be aware that food obtained from roadside stalls may not be properly cooked or refrigerated, and the same is true for some restaurants; not all of them adhere to the strict guidelines for safe food handling, food preparation, and hygiene.

- Meals containing chicken, undercooked hamburgers, raw sea-food, milk, or mayonnaise are highly suspect.
- Melons sold by weight are sometimes injected with contaminated water to increase their weight and should be avoided.
- Fruit juices are often prepared by unsanitary techniques and diluted with water.
- Raw vegetables, particularly lettuce, which is frequently fertilized with human feces, should not be consumed without washing it in a chlorine solution.

Mariners provisioning a boat in foreign ports can significantly extend the life of most produce and reduce the risk of food-borne infection by washing the produce in a bucket of bleach solution (15 mL of bleach per 3.75 L of water [1 tablespoon of bleach per gallon of water]), and then drying it with a clean towel. Soak the produce in diluted bleach or even dish soap for 20 minutes before rinsing and eating it. (You don't taste the soap any more than you would after you wash and rinse a glass or dish.)

Purchase unrefrigerated eggs, store them in their carton in a cool spot, and turn the carton over (180 degrees) twice a week; the eggs will keep for weeks.

Dishes and eating utensils can also be sources of contamination; they should be washed with drinking-quality water. Disinfect tap water used for brushing teeth, and practice good personal hygiene with frequent and thorough hand washing together with proper food-handling techniques.

Frequent hand washing with antibacterial/antiviral soaps helps to prevent spreading infections. Everyone should use soap and water before eating and after every bowel movement, and air-dry the hands. Alcohol-based and waterless hand cleansers are self-drying and require no towel, so they are excellent for use on a boat. Stay out of the camp kitchen or galley if ill, and do not handle group serving spoons and group food platters. Remember the rule of F's, which covers the modes of transmission of food-borne illness: food, fingers, fluids, and feces.

Antibiotics are not recommended for prevention of traveler's diarrhea but are reserved for treatment if sickness occurs, to limit the duration and severity of illness. Bismuth subsalicylate (Pepto-Bismol, Kaopectate) is effective in preventing diarrhea in about 60 percent of travelers, but must be taken in large quantities. Take 60 mL (4 tablespoons) four times a day, or 2 tablets four times a day, are needed. Unfortunately, this equates to a large amount of aspirin and can give some people stomach problems.

Signs and Symptoms

Symptoms usually begin abruptly 2 to 3 days after ingesting contaminated food or water. The diarrhea can be watery or soft, and there can be cramps, nausea, vomiting, malaise, and fever. Some strains of bacteria are more virulent and can spread through the body, causing kidney failure and occasionally death.

Treatment

1. See "Diarrhea: Treatment," page 172.
2. Antibiotics are effective for treating most cases of traveler's diarrhea. The best antibiotics are ciprofloxacin (Cipro) 500 mg twice a day for 3 to 5 days, levofloxacin (Levaquin) 500 mg daily for 3 days, or azithromycin (Zithromax) 250 mg once a day for 2 to 3 days. Ciprofloxacin and levofloxacin are not approved for use in children and may cause joint pain. A single dose of ciprofloxacin 750 mg or azithromycin 1000 mg is also effective. In parts of Southeast Asia, such as Thailand, bacterial resistance to ciprofloxacin is common, and azithromycin is recommended. Before traveling, consult the CDC website for updates regarding recommended treatment in the areas you may be visiting.

Giardiasis (Giardia)

Giardia is a hardy parasite that can thrive even in very cold water. Just one glass of contaminated water is enough to produce illness. Symptoms of giardiasis are usually delayed for 7 to 10 days after drinking contaminated water and may last 2 months or longer if the infection is not treated.

Signs and Symptoms

- Onset is usually gradual, with two to five loose or mushy stools per day.

- Stools smell foul and contain mucus.
- The person usually experiences a rumbling or gurgling feeling in the stomach, has foul-smelling gas, cramping abdominal pain, and nausea, and burps that taste like rotten eggs.
- General malaise and weight loss can occur.

Treatment

One of the following options will address the infection; alternative drugs will require a written prescription:

1. *Nitazoxanide (Alinia):* The dose for adults is 500 mg twice a day for 3 days. The dose for children is 100 mg twice a day for 3 days.
2. *Metronidazole (Flagyl):* The adult dose is 250 mg three times a day for 7 days. The pediatric dose is 5 mg per kilogram (1 kg = 2.2 pounds) of body weight per dose, three times per day, for 5 days. As with all medications for infants and children, it is best to consult a pediatrician.
3. *Tinidazole (Tiniba):* Can be taken as a single 2 g dose in adults to cure the infection.

Cryptosporidiosis (Crypto)

Cryptosporidium is a microscopic parasite similar to *Giardia* that lives in the feces of infected humans and animals. It is found in nearly all surface waters that have been tested in the United States. *Cryptosporidium* is a resilient parasite. It is not killed by chlorine or iodine at concentrations normally used to disinfect drinking water, and it can slip through many water filters. The parasite is between 2 and 5 microns in size; as a result, filters must be able to remove particles smaller than 2 microns to be effective in eliminating *Cryptosporidium* from the water supply. Fortunately, the bug is vulnerable to heat and can be killed simply by bringing water to a full boil.

Signs and Symptoms

In most healthy people, cryptosporidiosis causes abdominal cramps, low-grade fever, nausea, vomiting, and diarrhea, which can result in dehydration. Symptoms usually begin 2 to 7 days after drinking contaminated water and can last for 2 to 3 weeks before resolving on its own.

For people with AIDS, on chemotherapy, or with a weakened immune system, cryptosporidiosis may last for months and can be fatal.

Treatment
Nitazoxanide (Alinia) 500 mg twice a day for 3 days. Loperamide (Imodium) may help decrease fluid loss and intestinal cramping.

URINARY TRACT PROBLEMS
Bladder Infection
While a bladder infection is not usually a serious disease, it is very uncomfortable and, if untreated, it can spread to the kidneys and produce a potentially dangerous kidney infection.

Women are much more likely to develop a urinary tract infection than men, because the tube (urethra) that drains the bladder in women is much shorter. The short female urethra allows infection-causing bacteria a shorter, easier trip to the bladder, where they can multiply and produce an infection.

Prevention
- Drink plenty of fluids, to maintain a clear-looking urine.
- After going to the bathroom, women should wipe themselves from front to back to avoid contaminating the urethral entrance with bacteria from the bowels.
- Don't postpone urinating when you feel the urge to go. On a boat, be sure you have access to a toilet; on a river trip, go ashore. In any case, don't hold it in; frequent voiding prevents bacteria from multiplying and causing infection.
- Urinate immediately after sexual intercourse. This helps flush out any bacteria that may have accidentally been pushed into the urethra.
- In hot or humid conditions, wear loose-fitting pants and wipe the perineal area frequently with moist hygienic towelettes.
- Drinking cranberry juice may help prevent bladder infections. Cranberry juice appears to inhibit the adherence of certain bacteria to bladder cells. Unfortunately, other fruit juices have not been found to share this medicinal quality.

Signs and Symptoms
- Burning pain upon urination
- Urgent need to urinate frequently
- Cloudy, bloody, or bad-smelling urine
- Dull pain in lower abdomen

Treatment
Most bladder infections can be treated with a 3-day course of antibiotics, such as cephalexin (Keflex), amoxicillin clavulanate (Augmentin), or levofloxacin (Levaquin). The commonly used sulfa drugs (sulfonamide) increase the risk of severe sunburn and are best avoided in the boating environment. Another prescription drug, phenazopyridine (Pyridium) will help relieve pain and bladder spasms. It also turns urine and other body fluids reddish-orange, so don't wear expensive underclothes while taking it. Drink lots of fluid, especially cranberry juice if available.

Kidney Infection (Pyelonephritis)
Signs and Symptoms
Symptoms may include those for bladder infection with the addition of back pain in the flanks, fever, chills, nausea, or vomiting.

Treatment
1. Initially, treatment is the same as for bladder infections.
2. Obtain medical consultation or evacuate if high fever, chills, and lower back pain persist despite antibiotic treatment.

Kidney Stones
Stones form in the kidney when the urine becomes too concentrated. This is commonly caused by dehydration. If a stone passes out of the kidney, it can become lodged in the tubes leading to the bladder (ureters). Severe pain, blood in the urine, and infection may ensue.

Signs and Symptoms
- Intense waves of pain radiate from the lower back to the flank and lower abdomen, and occasionally to the groin.

- The person often rolls from side to side to find a more comfortable position (with appendicitis or other abdominal infections, the person usually lies still, because movement increases the pain).
- Other symptoms and signs include nausea, vomiting, an urge to urinate, and blood in the urine. The urine may turn red or brown and contain tiny clots.
- If infection is also present, symptoms may include shaking chills and fever.

Treatment

1. Drink plenty of fluids—at least 4 L (1 gallon) a day—which may help to flush out the stone and prevent new stones from forming.
2. Administer pain medication. An excellent medication for kidney stone pain is ibuprofen (Advil, Motrin). Narcotics, such as acetaminophen with hydrocodone (Vicodin), may be required.
3. Most kidney stones will eventually pass on their own. Occasionally, kidney stones can lead to infection and damage to the kidney.
4. Small stones may move and lodge, but still remain in lower portions of the urinary tract with spontaneous resolution of pain; therefore, follow up with a physician to be sure the stone has been passed.
5. Administer antibiotics (see "Kidney Infection [Pyelonephritis]," page 179) if infection is suspected.

Urinary Retention and Catheterization of the Urinary Bladder

All of the drugs used to prevent seasickness increase the risk of urinary retention (inability to pass urine). Men with enlarged prostate glands are especially susceptible to this problem, because the drugs interfere with the normal muscle function of the urinary bladder (and prostate), making it more difficult to void. If a man knows he has an enlarged prostate or if he has any of the following symptoms, he should consult his physician before taking seasickness medication, or at least try those meds while on land. While at sea, discontinue these drugs at the first sign of a problem.

The early signs and symptoms of urinary retention are decreased force of the urine stream, dribbling, difficulty starting the stream, a feeling of incomplete bladder emptying, lower abdominal pain, and frequent voiding of small amounts of urine. The person may suddenly be unable to void, with no warning. With complete obstruction, the bladder becomes enlarged and tender over the lowest middle area of the abdomen, above the pubic bone. Blunt trauma to the groin and a fractured pelvis may also quickly produce this condition. Obtain medical consultation before catheterizing these persons.

If urinary retention persists for more than a few hours, catheterization of the bladder is necessary. The catheter should be left inserted until the drug effects wear off (up to 48 hours). If the condition is unrelated to medication, the catheter should be left in place until medical consultation is obtained. Although urethral catheterization is considered a semi-sterile procedure, the body will tolerate a small amount of contamination as long as

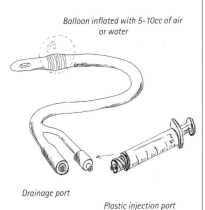

Balloon inflated with 5-10cc of air or water

Drainage port

Plastic injection port

Fig. 68

Continued on next page

Continued from previous page

the procedure is done as cleanly as possible. In any case, do your best to maintain sterile conditions. Having someone assist with the procedure will make it much easier. Wear clean medical exam gloves. If gloves are not available, then wash hands in warm, soapy water and perform the procedure with bare hands. Have a large container (1 L or 1 quart glass or bottle) and a 10- to 20-cc syringe ready to inflate the catheter balloon (**Fig. 68**). To insert the catheter in a male, follow this procedure:

1. Have the person lie faceup.
2. Put on clean or sterile gloves (see "How to Put On Surgical Gloves," page 68) and use the paper containing the gloves for a sterile work area. You can also use the larger sterile drape from the surgical kit.
3. Have the assistant open a packet of sterile lubricant and squirt it onto the paper, taking care not to touch the sterile field. Then have the person open and drop (or shake out) two antiseptic swabs, without touching them, onto the paper. The assistant now can carefully peel back the Foley catheter packaging, exposing the sterile catheter (or the inner package); the person wearing the gloves removes and places the catheter on the sterile field.
4. Elevate the penis with the gloved nondominant hand (if the person is uncircumcised, retract the foreskin); wipe the tip (the opening of the urethra) and the head of the penis with an antiseptic pad using the gloved dominant hand; use a circular motion, working outward from the urethral opening. Discard the cleansing pad away from the sterile field. Repeat this procedure with the second swab.
5. Instruct the person to relax and breathe deeply as you begin to insert the catheter. He will feel pressure as the catheter is being advanced.
6. Pick up the catheter with the gloved dominant hand, about 10 to 15 cm (4 to 6 inches) from the catheter tip, and swirl it around in the lubricant.
7. Lift up the lubricated end of the catheter and have the assistant pick up and touch only the opposite end (where the catheter drains and the balloon is inflated). This draining end, which is no longer sterile, should be held over the container to catch the urine.

8. Hold the penis perpendicular to the person's body with slight tension. Gently insert the lubricated tip of the catheter into the urethra while stretching and straightening the penis with the left hand. Slowly advance the catheter, usually 15 to 20 cm (6 to 8 inches), until urine begins to flow.

9. If you encounter resistance as you advance the catheter, slightly increase your traction on the penis and ask the person to cough or bear down as if to pass urine to help relax the entrance to the bladder; gently maneuver the catheter to advance it. Maintain steady gentle pressure but do not force it.

10. When the catheter tip enters the bladder, urine will flow continuously. Advance it about another 5 cm (2 inches), and have the assistant slowly inflate the balloon with the syringe using 10 cc sterile water, bottled water, or air inserted through the plastic injection port. Write down the amount you inserted.

11. If resistance or pain is felt while inflating the balloon, remove the air or fluid back into the syringe, and further advance the catheter, then attempt to reinflate the balloon. Never inflate the balloon until urine flow is established.

12. Once the balloon is inflated, pull back on the catheter until you feel resistance. This will anchor the catheter in the bladder and prevent it from sliding out.

13. If urine does not start flowing freely from the catheter, it is sometimes obstructed by lubricant or a small blood clot. Urine can flow by waiting a minute or two for the lubricant to dissolve or by aspiration of the drainage port with an empty syringe. Attach the drainage end of the catheter to an appropriate drainage bag. If a drainage bag is not available, the catheter can be taped to a bottle or plastic container and placed in a pocket or taped to the leg.

14. No antibiotics are necessary while the catheter is indwelling and draining. If antibiotics are available, it is a good idea to start them just prior to removal of the catheter and continue them for 48 hours. Ciprofloxacin (Cipro) 500 mg twice a day, levofloxacin (Levaquin) 500 mg daily, or amoxicillin clavulanate (Augmentin) 875 mg three times a day can be used.

15. When removing the catheter, the balloon must be deflated by gently withdrawing the amount of previously injected air or water (according to your notes) from the injection port.

GYNECOLOGICAL EMERGENCIES

Vaginal Bleeding

Female travelers may experience a change in their menstrual cycle due to stress and the rigors of a trip. It is important to differentiate irregular vaginal bleeding or cessation of vaginal bleeding from pregnancy. If there is any chance of pregnancy, test with a pregnancy test kit, using the first morning urine; the test is 99 percent accurate the first day of a missed period. Any abnormal bleeding or abdominal pain accompanied by vaginal bleeding that is not associated with a normal menstrual period should be evaluated by a physician immediately. An ectopic, or tubal, pregnancy should be suspected if a menstrual period has been missed and vaginal bleeding and pelvic cramps develop. The condition can rapidly become life-threatening if not treated.

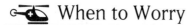 # When to Worry

Vaginal Bleeding
In a woman who is of childbearing age, any lower abdominal pain that is accompanied by vaginal bleeding and is not typical of a normal menstrual period should be evaluated for a possible ectopic pregnancy (abnormal pregnancy in the Fallopian tube). If a urine pregnancy test is negative, this condition is very unlikely.

Pelvic Infection

Signs and Symptoms

Pelvic pain associated with fever, chills, nausea, vomiting, and weakness may indicate a pelvic infection (uterus and ovaries). The lower abdomen is usually tender. A yellow-green vaginal discharge may be present also.

Treatment

If immediate medical care is not available, start oral antibiotics: doxycycline (Vibramycin) 100 mg twice a day, or levofloxacin (Levaquin) 500 mg daily together with metronidazole (Flagyl) 500 mg four times a day.

Vaginitis
Signs and Symptoms
If a vaginal discharge is white and creamy (like cottage cheese) and is associated with vaginal itching, and burning or pain on urination, it is usually vaginitis from a yeast infection.

Treatment
Vaginitis can be treated with a single dose of fluconazole (Diflucan) 150 mg taken orally (recommended treatment), or miconazole (Monistat) or clotrimazole Gyne-Lotrimin (Lotrimin) vaginal tablets (for 7 days) or cream (for 14 days). If none of these drugs is available, a vinegar douche can be helpful, as is airing the vaginal area and switching to cotton underwear or none at all. Changing into dry clothing after swimming, and avoiding tight-fitting underwear and tight pants, which prevent ventilation and drying in hot and humid weather, can often prevent yeast infections. If the discharge is frothy, white-gray, and accompanied by abdominal pain and fever, it is often due to trichomoniasis. Treat with metronidazole (Flagyl) 500 mg, 2 tablets twice for 1 day, or 4 tablets all at once as a single-dose treatment.

MILD ALLERGIC REACTIONS
Mild allergic reactions can occur as a result of insect stings, stings from hazardous marine life, food allergies, medications, exposure to animals, and other unknown reasons. (For severe allergic reactions, see "Anaphylactic Shock," page 37). Allergic reactions to insect stings are usually from the sting of a bee, wasp, hornet, yellow jacket, or fire ant. (See Insect and Anthropod Bites and Stings," page 188).

Signs and Symptoms
Often one may only develop hives (red raised skin welts) and itching without wheezing or other breathing problems.

Treatment
Mild allergic reactions may be managed with an antihistamine, such as diphenhydramine (Benadryl). The adult dose is 25 to 50 mg every 4 to 6 hours. The major side effect of this medication is drowsiness.

ASTHMA

Asthma, a respiratory disease involving the bronchial tubes in the lung, can be life-threatening, especially in children. Many factors can predispose a susceptible individual to an attack, including pollen, animal hair, certain foods, upper respiratory infections, emotional stress, exercise, or exposure to cold air.

Signs and Symptoms

During an acute attack, the muscles around the small breathing tubes in the lungs tighten or constrict, causing wheezing, coughing, and the sensation of not being able to get enough air (air hunger). Other signs of a severe attack include bluish tinge (cyanosis) to the lips and fingers, rapid heartbeat, gasping for air, and confusion.

Treatment

Breathing medications that contain bronchodilators (e.g., albuterol inhalers) are most helpful during an attack, because they are fast-acting. If the attack is severe, epinephrine from an EpiPen may be administered (see "Anaphylactic Shock," page 37). Other useful medications include diphenhydramine (Benadryl) 50 mg and prednisone (Deltasone and others). An adult should be given prednisone 60 mg orally if quick transfer to a medical facility is unlikely and the attack continues in severity; this dose could be reduced by 10 mg every third day until tapered completely (e.g., 60, 60, 50, 50, 40, 40). Before leaving on a trip with youngsters, discuss drug and dose regimens with their pediatrician or physician.

ALCOHOL WITHDRAWAL

Sailors often voluntarily or unexpectedly abstain from drinking alcohol when embarking on an ocean trip or offshore race. Weather conditions, watch schedules, or the rigors of sailing may preclude the usual cocktail hour; seasickness may decrease the desire to drink. For people who regularly consume alcohol on a daily basis, this sudden cessation may cause minor or major withdrawal symptoms.

Prevention

Crew members with a history of heavy alcohol consumption should consult their physician and abstain from alcohol at least a week before departure.

Signs and Symptoms

Alcohol is a brain depressant; abrupt withdrawal unmasks overactivity of the nervous system (similar to a rush of adrenaline). Minor withdrawal symptoms, starting as early as 6 to 8 hours after the last drink, include insomnia, tremors, palpitations (racing heartbeat), mild anxiety, headache, sweating, and loss of appetite. Improvement is gradual over 24 to 48 hours.

Treatment

Treat by administering diazepam (Valium) 5 to 10 mg every 4 to 6 hours, or lorazepam (Ativan) 1 to 2 mg every 4 to 6 hours, as needed to calm the person and prevent progression to major withdrawal symptoms. Continue medication until the person feels completely normal.

Some people experience hallucinations (usually visual), which rapidly clear within a day or two. Persons with a long history of chronic alcoholism can suffer seizures within 48 hours after their last drink and may develop an illness called delirium tremens (DTs) after 48 to 96 hours of abstinence. DTs includes striking mental status changes with hallucinations and disorientation, together with fever, severe agitation, sweating, vomiting, fever, rapid heart rate, and high blood pressure. Both hallucinations and DTs require evacuation and care in a medical facility.

Restraint and observation during withdrawal may be necessary to prevent injury, such as falling out of the bunk. Whenever possible, place the person withdrawing in a quiet, protective environment.

The administration of diazepam (Valium), 5 to 10 mg every 4 to 6 hours or more frequently, will help to calm the person prior to transfer. Keep a careful record of the amount administered. Alcohol should not be used as therapy for acute alcohol withdrawal.

INSECT AND ARTHROPOD BITES AND STINGS

Venom from insects can produce severe allergic reactions and lead to life-threatening anaphylactic shock (see "Anaphylactic Shock," page 37). More commonly, insect bites and stings are painful and produce local reactions (redness, swelling) at the site.

General Treatment

1. Ice or cold packs will help alleviate local pain and swelling.
2. Sting-relief swabs may help relieve pain when applied topically, as can aloe vera gel.
3. Oral antihistamines, such as diphenhydramine (Benadryl) 25 to 50 mg every 4 hours, are helpful in relieving the itching, rash, and swelling associated with many insect bites and stings.
4. The principles of wound care (see "Managing Wounds," page 119) apply to bites and stings as well. Any bite or sting can become infected and should therefore be examined at regular intervals for progressive redness, swelling, pain, or pus drainage.
5. Infectious diseases can be spread by insect bites, especially in tropical and developing countries. Wearing protective clothing and applying insect repellents containing DEET are important preventive measures (see "Lyme Disease," page 196, and "Malaria," page 288).

Bee Stings

Honeybees leave a stinger and venom sac in the person after a sting. Hornets, yellow jackets, bumblebees, and wasps do not leave a stinger and may puncture a person repeatedly.

Signs and Symptoms

Pain is immediate and may be accompanied by swelling, redness, and warmth at the site.

Treatment

1. If anaphylactic shock occurs, it must be treated immediately with epinephrine and antihistamines (see "Anaphylactic Shock," page 37).

2. After a honeybee sting, first remove the stinger and venom sac as quickly as possible. Even with the rest of the bee gone, the venom sac can continue to pump venom into your skin. Do not hesitate or fumble for a pocketknife or credit card to scrape the stinger out of the skin. It is better to grab the stinger and yank it out quickly than to worry about pinching or squeezing more venom from the sac.
3. Apply ice or cold water to the sting site.
4. Anesthetic sprays, swabs, and creams may help relieve pain.
5. For adults, administer 25 to 50 mg diphenhydramine (Benadryl) for progressive itching, swelling, or redness.

☀ Weiss Advice

Taking the Sting Out of Bee and Wasp Venom

For bee venom (which is acid), apply a paste of baking soda and water. For wasp venom (which is alkaline), apply vinegar, lemon juice, or another acidic substance. Meat tenderizer applied locally to the sting site may also be effective in denaturing the venom and relieving pain and inflammation.

Black Widow Spider Bites

Black widow spiders *(Lactrodectus mactans)* are about 1.6 cm (⁵⁄₈-inch–long and black with a red hourglass mark on the underside of the abdomen **(Fig. 69)**. They like to hang out in woodpiles, stone walls, and outhouses. They generally are nocturnal.

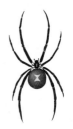

Signs and Symptoms

The black widow's bite feels like a sharp pinprick but sometimes may go unnoticed. Within an hour, the person may develop a tingling and numbing sensation in the palms of the hands and bottoms of the feet, along with muscle

Fig. 69 *Black widow spider*

cramps, particularly in the abdomen (stomach) and back. In severe cases, the stomach muscles may become rigid and boardlike. Sweating and vomiting are common, and the person may complain of headache and weakness. High blood pressure and seizures can occur.

Treatment
Most people will recover in 8 to 12 hours without treatment. Small children and elderly persons, however, may have severe reactions, occasionally leading to death.

1. Apply ice packs to the bite to relieve pain.
2. Transport the person to a medical facility as soon as possible.
3. Muscle relaxers such as diazepam (Valium) or lorazepam (Ativan) will help relieve muscle spasms.
4. A specific antidote is available for those suffering severe symptoms.

Brown Recluse Spider Bites
The brown recluse spider *(Loxosceles reclusa)* is found most commonly in the South and southern Midwest regions of the United States. The spider is brownish, with a body length of just under 10 mm ($^1/_2$ inch). A characteristic dark violin-shaped marking is found on the top of the upper section of the body (**Fig. 70**).

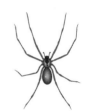

Fig. 70 *Brown recluse spider*

Signs and Symptoms
The bite sensation is initially mild, producing the same degree of pain as that of an ant sting. The stinging subsides over 6 to 8 hours and is replaced by aching and itching at the bite site. Within 1 to 5 hours, a painful red blister appears, surrounded by a bull's-eye of whitish-blue discoloration. Over the next 10 to 14 days the blister ruptures and a gradually enlarging ulcer crater develops, with further destruction of tissue. Fever, chills, weakness, nausea, and vomiting may develop within 24 to 48 hours of the bite.

Treatment
1. Apply ice or cold compresses to the wound for pain relief.
2. If the blister has ruptured, apply a topical antibiotic ointment to the wound and cover with a nonadherent sterile dressing and bandage.

3. Anyone bitten should obtain medical care as soon as possible. An antivenin is now available, which, when used early, can prevent loss of tissue and scarring.

Tarantula Bites

Tarantulas are large, slow spiders that sometimes bite.

Signs and Symptoms

The bite of a tarantula can be painful and can sometimes become infected.

Treatment

1. Apply ice for pain relief.
2. Elevate and immobilize the bitten extremity to reduce pain.
3. Apply an antibiotic ointment to the site.
4. Take ibuprofen (Advil, Motrin) or acetaminophen (Tylenol) for pain and antihistamines for itching.

Scorpion Stings

Scorpions are nocturnal, hiding during the day under bark, in rocky crevices, or in the sand. They are frequently found along riverbank campsites; however, scorpions are found in virtually every terrestrial habitat.

Prevention

Stings can be avoided by shaking out your shoes or boots and clothes in the morning before dressing, not walking barefoot after dark, and looking before picking up rocks or wood.

Signs and Symptoms

Most North American scorpion stings produce only localized pain and swelling. The stinger in the scorpion's tail injects the venom. The pain of a nonlethal species is similar to that of a wasp or hornet, and the treatment is similar. Severe allergic reactions to scorpion stings are rare.

The potentially lethal scorpion found in the United States is *Centruroides sculpturatus,* also known as the bark scorpion due to its habit of hiding beneath loose and fallen pieces of tree bark. It is found in the desert areas of the southwestern United States (Arizona, California,

New Mexico, and Texas) and northern Mexico. The bark scorpion is frequently found along sandy riverbanks, so paddlers should be vigilant in riverside campsites. It is usually small (2 to 4 cm [1 to 2 inches] in length), and straw-yellow colored, with long slender pincers, as opposed to bulky and lobsterlike. The venom contains neurotoxins that can be lethal, but usually only in infants or small children.

The bark scorpion's sting causes immediate pain, which is worsened by tapping lightly over the bite site. Other symptoms include restlessness, muscle twitching that can sometimes look like a seizure, blurred vision, roving eye movements, trouble swallowing, drooling, slurred speech, difficulty breathing, and numbness and tingling around the mouth, feet, and hands.

Treatment

1. Place a piece of ice over the sting area to reduce pain.
2. Seek professional medical care as soon as possible, as an antivenin is available in the areas where lethal scorpions live.

Fire Ant Bites

Fire ants (Solenopsis invicta) are found in the southeastern states, Texas, and parts of California. They range in color from dull yellow to red or black. The ants are tenacious, and swarm and sting a person repeatedly.

Signs and Symptoms

Initially, a cluster of small painful and itchy blisters develops, which usually evolves into small pustules (boils) within 24 hours. The skin over the pustules will slough away in 2 to 3 days, after which the sores heal. Some persons develop a severe reaction characterized by large red swollen welts that are very itchy. About 1 percent of stings are followed by severe allergic reactions.

Treatment

1. Apply ice or cold packs to the area. Topical sting-relief swabs help relieve the pain.
2. Administer ibuprofen (Advil, Motrin) or acetaminophen (Tylenol) with codeine for pain.

3. The rash and itching can be treated with antihistamines, such as diphenhydramine (Benadryl) 25 to 50 mg every 4 to 6 hours. Topical steroid creams, such as betamethasone valerate (Valisone 0.1%) or triamcinolone may also help to reduce the itching. In severe cases, prepackaged methylprednisolone (Medrol Dosepak), set up for daily tapering of dose, or prednisone (Deltasone and others) 40 to 60 mg orally initially and then tapered, will dramatically reduce itching.

Stinging Caterpillars

The puss caterpillar or woolly slug *(Megalopyge opercularis)*, found in the southern United States, has venomous bristles that inflict a painful sting.

Signs and Symptoms

Contact with one causes instant pain, followed by redness and swelling at the site. Symptoms usually subside within 24 hours. In rare cases, nausea, headache, fever, vomiting, and shock may occur.

Treatment

1. Pat the skin with a piece of adhesive tape to remove any remaining bristles.
2. Apply hydrocortisone cream to the site to reduce itching, or take an oral antihistamine such as diphenhydramine (Benadryl).

Tick Bites

Ticks reach out from vegetation (usually tall blades of grass) with their front legs and attach to people and animals as they pass by. Once a tick lands on a person, it clings to hair or clothing and waits for several hours until the individual is at rest. Then it moves to an exposed area, often around the tops of the socks or at the neckline, attaches itself, and begins feeding. An anesthetic agent in the tick's saliva usually makes the bite painless. Ticks feed from 2 hours to several days before dropping off.

Ticks secrete saliva and disease-producing organisms into the host while feeding. About a hundred tick species transmit infections to man. The most infamous are the tiny deer tick *(Ixodes scapularis)* and the black-legged tick *(Ixodes pacificus)*. Both are capable of causing Lyme disease, ehrlichiosis, and babesiosis. The tiny nymph (the size of a poppy seed) and adult (the size of a sesame seed) both transmit these diseases, most frequently in the late spring and summer. Bites from the Rocky Mountain wood tick *(Dermacentor andersoni)* and dog tick *(Dermacentor variabilis)* can cause Rocky Mountain spotted fever and tularemia; the lone star tick *(Amblyomma americanum)* is also a vector for tularemia as well as ehrlichiosis. Because of the many diseases associated with ticks, seek medical treatment for any illness (especially one with fever, chills, rash, and headache) following a tick bite. If possible, wrap the tick in a piece of paper or tape and save it for identification.

Prevention
- Spray tents, sleeping bags, and clothing with permethrin, an insecticide that kills ticks before they have a chance to get embedded in your skin. Permethrin remains effective on clothing for up to 2 weeks, and through several washings. Concentrate the application on the lower hem, cuffs, and neckline of clothing. Use it on companionway screens and mosquito netting. It should not be used directly on the skin.
- Apply an insect repellent with DEET to your skin.
- Check yourself and your companions for ticks ("tick patrol") at least every 4 hours when in tick country.
- Wear long pants that are tucked into the socks.
- Wear clothing that is light in color, making it easier to spot ticks.
- Be especially vigilant for ticks (especially those causing Lyme disease) in tall grasses along the seashore, the banks of rivers, lakes, and estuaries, and wooded areas with heavy underbrush frequented by deer.
- Be alert for symptoms of tick-borne diseases with or without evidence of a tick bite.
- It takes about 3 days (72 hours) for a feeding tick to suck blood and transmit the spirochete. If you remove the tick the same day it bites you, infection is unlikely. Ticks not engorged with blood and ones that remain unattached do not transmit disease. A single 200 mg dose of doxycycline (Vibramycin) given within 72 hours after a tick bite can prevent Lyme disease. It is recommended to treat any

one who removes an attached tick with 200 mg of doxycycline, since the time the tick has been on the person may not always be established with certainty. If the person has any fever, rash, headache, or any symptoms suggestive of Lyme disease, a full course of antibiotics is necessary. Doxycycline should not be used in children under 8 years old. Travelers in heavily infested areas might stock this prescription antibiotic in their medical kit.

Removing an Embedded Tick

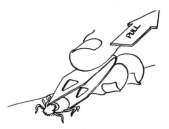

Fig. 71 *Removing a tick*

- Always wear protective gloves or use a barrier when handling engorged ticks.
- Grasp the tick as close to the skin or surface as possible with tweezers, taking care not to crush, squeeze, or puncture the body (**Fig. 71**). Apply steady, straight, upward traction to remove the tick. It may take a couple of minutes to convince the tick to let go. Avoid twisting, as the tick can break off and leave behind mouthparts.
- Do not try to remove anything left behind, as those pieces will eventually work themselves out.
- Clean the site with an antiseptic towelette, then apply a topical antibiotic.
- Traditional folk methods for removing ticks, such as applying fingernail polish, petrolatum jelly, rubbing alcohol, or a hot match, increase the chance that the tick will salivate or regurgitate into the wound, thus spreading infection.

Local Reactions

Tick bites can occasionally produce a painful red and swollen wound at the puncture site, which can take 1 or 2 weeks to heal. The site can also become infected, which will require topical and oral antibiotics.

Some ticks carry a neurotoxin in their saliva, and on rare occasions a bite can lead to a temporary, or sometimes fatal, paralysis. Paralysis usually occurs only after prolonged attachment (more than 5 days) and begins in the legs and spreads to the arms, trunk, and head. Removal of the tick stops the paralysis, and the person recovers completely within several hours.

Lyme Disease

Lyme disease is an infection caused by a spirochete, a type of bacteria that invades the body during the bite of an infected tick. Lyme disease is now the most common tick-transmitted infection. The majority of people with Lyme disease do not recall seeing or being bitten by the tick.

Lyme disease is most common in the Northeast (Connecticut, Maine, Massachusetts, New Jersey, New York, Pennsylvania, and Rhode Island), in the upper Midwest (especially Michigan, Minnesota, and Wisconsin), and on the Pacific coast (California and Oregon). In areas of the Northeast, 90 percent of the deer ticks are infected with Lyme disease. In the West, only 1 to 2 percent of the ticks are infected.

Signs and Symptoms

Ranging from 3 days to a month (average of 7 days) after the tick bite, 80 percent of infected individuals develop an expanding, circular red rash (erythema migrans). As the rash expands, it may form an irregularly shaped large red area, or more typically, it will appear as a bull's-eye with a central red spot surrounded by a halo of clear skin and an outer border of bright red skin. Sometimes the rash is doughnut-shaped, with clearing of the redness in the center. It spreads slowly, up to 2.5 cm (1 inch) daily, and may attain more than 30 cm (12 inches) in diameter. The rash may appear anywhere, unrelated to the bite site, although the thigh, groin, back, chest, and armpit are the most common locations. The rash is warm to the touch and usually described as itchy or burning, but it is rarely painful. The rash fades after an average of 28 days without treatment; with antibiotics, the rash resolves after several days.

Flu-like symptoms, such as fever, extreme fatigue, headache, and muscle and joint aches, may develop before or with the rash, and last for a few days.

About 20 percent of untreated people develop severe complications within weeks or months after the bite, ranging from heart and neurologic problems, such as paralysis of the muscle on one side of the face, to severe attacks of arthritis, with swelling and pain in the larger joints.

Treatment

If a red rash or flu-like symptoms are observed after a tick bite, medical attention should be obtained. Where Lyme disease is endemic, treatment should be started based on the clinical presentation (the signs and symptoms). Blood tests are negative early in the disease, and some laboratories may be unreliable. The standard treatment is 3 weeks of amoxicillin 500 mg three times daily, or doxycycline (Vibramycin) 100 mg twice daily for 3 weeks. (It is important to cover up to prevent excessive sunburn while using doxycycline.) Failure to improve after starting antibiotics may indicate that a person is suffering from two different tick diseases at the same time.

VENOMOUS SNAKEBITES

There are two classes of poisonous snakes in the United States:

- *Pit vipers* (rattlesnakes, water moccasins [cottonmouths], and copperheads) have a characteristic triangular head, a deep pit (heat receptor organ) between the eye and nostril, and a catlike, elliptical pupil.
- *Elapids* (coral snakes) are characterized by their color pattern with red, black, and yellow or white bands encircling the body. The fangs are short—these snakes bite by chewing rather than by striking.

All states except Alaska, Hawaii, and Maine are home to at least one species of venomous snake. States with a high incidence (10 or more hospitalizations per year) of venomous snakebites include Arkansas, Georgia, Louisiana, Mississippi, Texas, and West Virginia. Florida, Oklahoma, New Mexico, and South Carolina are closely approaching these figures.

About 90 percent of snakebites occur between April and October, because snakes are more active in warm months of the year. The chance of dying from a venomous snakebite in the wilderness is extremely remote—about 1 in 12 million.

Snakes can strike from up to one-half their body length away, and may bite and not inject venom (dry bite). No poisoning occurs in about 20 to 30 percent of rattlesnake bites, and fewer than 40 percent of coral snake bites.

Pit Viper Envenomation
Signs and Symptoms
- One or more fang marks (Rattlesnake bites may leave one, two, or even three fang marks.)
- Local, burning pain immediately after the bite
- Swelling at the site of the bite, usually beginning within 5 to 20 minutes and spreading slowly over a period of 6 to 12 hours (The faster the swelling progresses up the arm or leg, the worse the degree of envenomation.)
- Bruising (black-and-blue discoloration) and blister formation at the bite site
- Numbness and tingling of the lips and face, usually within 60 minutes after the bite
- Twitching of the muscles around the eyes and mouth
- Rubbery or metallic taste in the mouth
- After 6 to 12 hours, possible bleeding from the gums and nose
- Possible weakness, sweating, nausea, vomiting, and faintness

Treatment
The definitive treatment for snake-venom poisoning is the administration of antivenin. The most important aspect of therapy is to get the person to a medical facility as quickly as possible.
1. Rinse the area around the bite site with water to remove any venom that might remain on the skin.
2. Clean the wound and cover with a sterile dressing.
3. Remove any rings or jewelry.
4. Do not apply suction as first aid for snakebites. Suction has no benefit and may aggravate the injury. Do not make incisions over the bite to encourage bleeding.

5. Apply a pressure immobilization bandage around the entire length of the bitten extremity as soon as possible (**Fig. 72**). An elastic wrap bandage works best, but torn or cut strips of any flexible material, such as clothing or a towel, may be used. The wrap is started beyond the bite site and continued upward toward the torso in an even fashion, about as tightly as one would wrap a sprained ankle. The wrap should not be uncomfortable, and it should be loose enough to allow a finger to be slipped under it. Cut or take clothing off

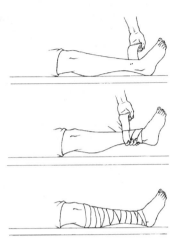

Fig. 72 *Application of a pressure immobilization bandage*

very gently, as the movement of doing so might promote the movement of venom into the bloodstream. Extend the bandage as high as possible up the limb, but leave the tips of the fingers or toes unbandaged to allow the circulation to be checked.

6. Immobilize the injured part as you would for a fracture, and allow it to lie just below the level of the heart. If the bite is on a hand or arm, also apply a sling.

7. Transport the person to the nearest hospital as soon as possible. So that antivenin can be located and procured, notify the facility that you are bringing in a snakebite victim.

8. It is not necessary to kill the snake and transport it for identification. If the snake is killed, it should not be directly handled, but it should be transported in a closed container.

CAUTION: Decapitated snake heads can still produce envenomation.

Things Not to Do for a Snakebite

1. Do not make any incisions in the skin or apply suction with your mouth.
2. Do not apply ice or a tourniquet.
3. Do not shock the person with a stun gun or electrical current.

Elapid (Coral Snake) Envenomation

Signs and Symptoms
- Burning pain at the site of the bite
- Numbness and/or weakness of a bitten arm or leg within 90 minutes
- Twitching, nervousness, drowsiness, increased salivation, and drooling within 1 to 3 hours
- Slurred speech, double vision, difficulty talking and swallowing, and difficulty breathing within 5 to 10 hours
- Possible total paralysis
- Possible delay of symptoms up to 13 hours after the bite

Treatment
1. Treatment is the same as for a pit viper bite.
2. Early use of the pressure immobilization technique is highly recommended (**Fig. 72**, page 199).

VENOMOUS LIZARDS

The Gila monster and the Mexican beaded lizard are found only in the Great Sonoran Desert area in southern Arizona and northwestern Mexico. Both possess venom glands and grooved teeth capable of envenomating humans. Not all bites result in envenomation, since the lizard may only nip the person or not expel any venom during a bite. Gila monsters may hang on tenaciously during a bite, and pliers or a sharp knife may be required to loosen the grip of its jaws.

Signs and Symptoms
- Pain and severe burning are felt at the wound site within 5 minutes and may radiate up the extremity. Intense pain may last from 3 to 5 hours and then subside after 8 hours.

■ Swelling occurs at the wound site, usually within 15 minutes, and progresses slowly up the extremity. Blue discoloration may appear around the wound.

Treatment
1. Clean the wound thoroughly as you would for any laceration (see "Managing Wounds," page 119).
2. Inspect the wound and remove any shed or broken teeth.
3. Immobilize and elevate the extremity.
4. Obtain medical care as soon as possible.

OTHER ANIMAL BITES

Human or animal bites, including marine animals (see "Hazardous Marine Life," page 264), often become infected and can transmit diseases, such as rabies. Cat bites are especially prone to infection.

General Treatment
1. Clean the wound vigorously (see "Managing Wounds," page 119).
2. The best antiseptic for bite wounds is benzalkonium chloride, because it helps to kill the rabies virus.
3. Never close an animal bite with sutures or tape. Pack the wound with saline-moistened gauze pads and cover with another dressing and bandage. Change the dressing daily.
4. Seek medical attention as soon as possible. If professional care is delayed for more than 12 hours, consider starting the oral antibiotic amoxicillin clavulanate (Augmentin) 875 mg twice daily for 7 or more days.

Rabies
Although rabies is uncommon, if not treated right away it will kill 100 percent of those bitten. In the United States, raccoons, skunks, and bats account for 96 percent of rabies cases, while foxes and coyotes are the culprits in most of the remaining cases. Any unprovoked attack by one of these animals should be considered an attack by a rabid animal.

Infection can occur even without a bite. The lick of an animal infected with rabies can transmit the disease if the saliva contacts an open wound or mucous membrane. People have become infected with rabies after breathing the virus in bat-ridden caves. Squirrels, rats, mice, gerbils, chipmunks, and opossums have not been found to transmit rabies.

The rabies virus, transmitted to humans in the saliva of infected animals, attaches itself to nerves at the bite site. It then moves along the nerves to the brain. The virus causes no reaction until it reaches the brain, so the infection goes unnoticed until then. Once the virus has invaded the brain and symptoms develop, treatment is no longer effective and death is inevitable.

The average time between the bite and the appearance of symptoms is 30 days. A bite on a leg allows more time for treatment than a bite on an arm, because the virus has farther to travel to reach the brain. Bites around the face are particularly dangerous and must be treated immediately.

Signs and Symptoms

The initial symptoms of rabies are nonspecific and include malaise, fatigue, anxiety, agitation, irritability, insomnia, fever, headache, nausea, vomiting, and sore throat. After 2 to 10 days, the person may become aggressive, hyperactive, irrational, and prone to seizures and hallucinations.

Treatment

1. Swab the wound aggressively and thoroughly with benzalkonium chloride. If it is unavailable, scrub the wound vigorously with soap and water. Then irrigate the wound with lots of water.
2. If the biting animal can be safely captured, it should be observed for signs of rabies. If it's killed, the brain tissue can be tested for the virus.
3. Anyone who has been bitten should seek the assistance of a physician as soon as possible. The doctor will determine the need for rabies vaccination. For persons previously unvaccinated with rabies vaccine, the CDC currently recommends a reduced regimen of 4 doses administered intramuscularly. The first dose of the

4-dose course should be administered as soon as possible after exposure (day 0). Additional doses then should be administered on days 3, 7, and 14 after the first vaccination. Anti-rabies serum must also be given.

SEASICKNESS

Seasickness *(mal de mer)* is the most common and significant medical illness for all mariners, whether boating in local home waters or offshore. It is, however, a self-limited condition, and symptoms subside as one acclimates over 2 to 3 days. The balance center's ability to adapt to new sea conditions is commonly called "getting your sea legs." Nearly everyone will develop seasickness with sufficient stimuli; however, individual susceptibility is enormously variable.

The underlying cause of seasickness involves a conflict of sensory input processed by the brain to orient the body's position. Someone inside the cabin of a heeling or rolling boat is inviting seasickness. Belowdecks, the eyes (the visual cue) are oriented to the floor and ceiling, and see no tilt from a vertical upright position. At the same time, fluid in the inner ear's motion sensors constantly shifts and sends a different message about position and movement to the brain's balance center. This mix of sensory data from the eyes and inner ear arrives in complex and conflicting combinations, creating a sensory conflict that activates the link between the balance center and the vomiting center in the brain. The balance brain initiates corrective eye, head, and body movement readily when on land but needs time to learn to anticipate the boat's motion in order to harmonize boat and body movement. As this happens, sensory conflict and seasickness disappear.

Prevention

Medication is much more effective in preventing symptoms than in reversing them. Therefore, seasickness medication should be administered a few hours before leaving port, or even the night prior to departure (see **Table 2**, page 204). Begin a trip well-hydrated and free of the aftereffects of alcohol, which impair vestibular function and sensitize the vestibular apparatus to any motion. Try to avoid alcohol completely for at least 6 to 12 hours before departure. No particular food or diet has been shown to prevent seasickness. Try to snack on bland foods throughout the day, to maintain energy levels until meals are regularly tolerated. Cheese and crackers, energy bars, fruit, trail mix, dry granola, candy, and popcorn work well. Sip drinks containing sugar and electrolytes, as found in a variety of sports drinks, throughout the day. It is essential to maintain hydration and some nutritional intake to avoid dehydration and low blood sugar. The body requires a minimum of 1.5 L (1.5 quarts of fluid a day; the symptoms of dehydration often mimic those of seasickness.

Table 2: Medications for Seasickness

Brand/Generic Name	Dose	Interval
Diphenhydramine/ Benadryl (OTC)	25–50 mg tablet	6–8 hrs.
Dimenhydrinate/ Dramamine (OTC)	50–100 mg tablet (max 400 mg/day)	4–6 hrs.
Meclizine/ Bonine (OTC)	12.5–25 mg tablet (max 100 mg/day)	6–8 hrs.
Cinnarizine/ Stugeron	15-mg tablet (max 100 mg/day)	6–12 hrs.
Scopolamine/ Transderm Scōp	1.5-mg skin patch	72 hrs.
Scopolamine/ Scopace	0.4-mg tablet (max 2.4 mg/day)	8 hrs.
Promethazine/ Phenergan	12.5–25–50 mg tablet, suppository, or intra-muscular (IM) injection	Variable intervals, depending on dose/ preparation

Ginger may be useful in individual cases. Ginger is readily available in 500 mg capsules and sold in marine stores as Sailors' Secret. The suggested dose is 1000 mg every 6 hours, starting 30 minutes prior to the trip; it is less effective when given to someone who is already nauseated. The capsules can be supplemented with foods containing lower concentrations of ginger, such as gingersnap cookies, ginger ale, or ginger tea, and candied ginger. Too much ginger may cause heartburn; people with gallstones should not take it, because it can provoke an attack of abdominal pain by stimulating the flow of bile.

Acupressure is useful for some people to prevent seasickness. However, some experts on space and motion sickness still consider acupressure no better than a placebo. For those who wish to avoid the use of medications, it is certainly worth a try. Pressure should be applied on the inside part of the forearm over the median nerve. This is found two to three fingerbreadths above the wrist joint between the two prominent finger flexor tendons. Elastic wrist straps with plastic studs that create pressure over this point are available commercially. Some boaters place one on each forearm.

Recommendations for preventing seasickness are directed toward reducing sensory conflict by limiting the time belowdecks while underway, especially early in the trip. This will help the eyes to see what "the ears are feeling." After departure, stay on deck and amidships or aft, where pitching and rolling are less severe. Obtain a broad view of the horizon using direct and peripheral (side) vision. This provides a stable and level point of reference. Peeking out of a porthole at the sky and water doesn't really help. Avoid close visual tasks such as prolonged reading, writing, and navigation. Avoid areas with fumes (especially diesel) and odors that can stimulate nausea. Try to prepare some meals ahead of time and have frequently used gear easily available to avoid prolonged time belowdecks. Continue medication at the suggested intervals; try tapering the dose after the first or second day.

Signs and Symptoms

The key to prevention is to recognize the earliest symptoms. These may include the following: yawning, sighing, dry mouth or salivating, drowsiness, headache, dizziness, and lethargy. Pallor, cold sweats, belching, nausea, and vomiting ensue. Some persons don't have these complaints but experience headache, apathy, and depression. The side effects of some seasickness medications mimic seasickness, creating a diagnostic dilemma. The window of opportunity for early intervention is often missed, because early signs are not recognized or the person is in denial about the condition.

At best, seasickness is moderately disabling. It can lead to rapid mental and physical deterioration marked by progressive dehydration, loss of manual dexterity, balance, judgment, and loss of the will to survive. Fatalities from seasickness have occurred because of poor seamanship and complications arising during hazardous and sometimes unnecessary emergency evacuations.

Seasickness impairs reasoning. Sailors often lose the ability to analyze and integrate complex data (weather charts, radar, etc.), which leads to impaired judgment and problem solving. Compounding this problem are the medications used to prevent or treat seasickness. Their side effects may include drowsiness, confusion, and loss of concentration.

Treatment

At the first sign of seasickness, one immediate remedy that works for most crew members is to take over the helm. The active mental and physical activity required to steer the ship, together with the visual focus on the horizon and waves, helps to reorient the body's equilibrium. Steer the boat by reference to clouds, the horizon, distant marks, and oncoming waves. Stand and feel the waves, posturing to anticipate the boat's motion by "riding" the waves. Wave riding synchronizes sensory input and expectations of motion. Keep head, shoulders, and upper body balanced over the hips; stay in balance; and gain postural control gracefully, as though the body were truly gimbaled on the deck. Sitting in the cockpit, one can still ride the waves, watch the horizon line, and anticipate the boat's motion by watching the oncoming waves. Postural anticipation of the boat's motion is the natural cure for seasickness.

Debilitated seasick crew can easily fall or be washed overboard. They should always wear a safety harness on deck and be closely monitored. When trying to sleep, the safest place is belowdecks in a secure, well-ventilated berth. If the body is fixed in a safe position, wedged in place to prevent rolling around, then rest and recovery can proceed.

Medications for seasickness are listed in **Table 2**, page 204. Promethazine (Phenergan) is useful for prophylactic and active treatment of seasickness and can be administered as a suppository, by deep intramuscular (IM) injection, and orally as a tablet or syrup. It is a very effective drug with some potential side effects, which should be reviewed with your physician. NASA astronauts use intramuscular promethazine.

Transdermal scopolamine (Transderm Scōp) is the most popular agent used for prevention of motion sickness. The drug is delivered via an adhesive patch placed behind the ear 6 or more hours before departure; the patch will last for up to 3 days, often with minimal side effects. The most common adverse effects are dry mouth, drowsiness, and urinary retention. Other undesirable side effects include blurred vision (which may persist for weeks), short-term memory loss, and problems denoted by the well-known mnemonic "hot as hell, dry as a bone, blind as a bat, mad as a hatter." Follow the directions carefully, and wash hands thoroughly after application, because temporary blurring of vision and dilation of the pupils may occur if the drug is on your fingers and comes in contact with the eyes. Apply only one patch at a time. Scopolamine (Transderm Scōp patch) is not recommended for children, persons with glaucoma (remove the patch immediately if eye pain occurs suddenly), and men with an enlarged prostate (it will cause urinary retention). Long-term (repeated and continuous) use may produce withdrawal symptoms such as nausea, dizziness, headache, and equilibrium disturbances.

Scopolamine in pill form (Scopace) is an alternative to the patch. The chief advantage is the dosing flexibility. The fixed dose from the patch may be excessive for small individuals and inadequate for larger people. Taking the lowest effective dose can minimize side effects. The current recommendation is 1 tablet (0.4 mg) or 2 tablets (0.8 mg) 1 hour prior to departure, and 1 to 2 tablets every 8 hours as needed thereafter.

The antihistamines meclizine (Bonine) and dimenhydrinate (Dramamine) are available over-the-counter (OTC), without prescription. They are effective for many sailors, as are the other prescription medications listed in **Table 2**. The popular antihistamine cinnarizine (Stugeron) is not sold in the United States but is available OTC in Europe, Bermuda, Canada, and Mexico, and it can be obtained legally from online Canadian pharmacies. Many sailors favor it, because it is less sedating than all other antihistamines and has fewer reported side effects.

Side effects of all the antihistamines include drowsiness, dry mouth, blurred vision, irritability, urinary retention, dizziness, and headache. Meclizine is thought to cause less drowsiness and confusion. Antihistamines cause thickened bronchial secretions and should be used with caution in people with asthma. An effective nonprescription drug to counteract drowsiness is the decongestant pseudoephedrine (Sudafed), which is available in 30 to 100 mg doses; caffeine 200 mg is also useful and may potentiate the beneficial effects of promethazine (Phenergan). The newer generation of nonsedating long-acting antihistamines (e.g., ceterizine [Zyrtec]) are ineffective in preventing seasickness. Ondansetron (Zofran) is very effective for treatment of nausea and vomiting caused by many different conditions. It is manufactured as an oral disintegrating tablet. Unfortunately, ondansetron does not prevent seasickness.

All therapies are subject to the placebo effect, and no well-controlled trials have compared and evaluated different treatments. Many products cite only testimonials. The protection conferred by drugs is a matter of degree; there is no magic bullet to prevent seasickness in everyone. It is not uncommon for one drug in a category (e.g., antihistamine) to be effective and a related drug to provide no benefit; the same is true for side effects. Evaluate medication side effects before boating. Experiment with drugs onshore, and take a few doses at the recommended intervals for a day or more. Find a drug that works best for you with minimal side effects and stick with it. If all else fails, follow Samuel Johnson's eighteenth-century advice: "To cure seasickness, find a good big oak tree and wrap your arms around it."

ILLNESSES CAUSED BY COLD

Cold environments present a wide range of potential injuries and illnesses for boaters unprepared to protect themselves and the crew from heat loss and cold-induced physical injury; the consequences range from possible loss of limbs to loss of life. The following sections on cold injury deal with this serious environmental threat to safety, health, and survival.

Frostnip, Frostbite, and Immersion Foot

Prevention

Frostbite occurs in cold and windy weather conditions. Even if the temperature outdoors is not very cold, high winds can reduce the effective temperature to a dangerously low level. The chilling effect of air at 20°F moving at 64 km/h (40 miles per hour) is the same as –20°F air on a still day.

On long trips it is important to drink sufficient fluids to prevent dehydration and provide fuel (food) for your body to generate heat. If the body is cold and dehydrated, it will shunt (redirect) blood away from the skin, predisposing you to frostbite.

Other predisposing factors to frostbite include smoking, tight clothing and shoes, and contact of bare flesh with cold metal. Individuals with diabetes, known sensitivity to cold, and poor circulation are more likely to suffer frostbite.

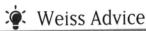 Weiss Advice

Windmilling for Warmth

If you feel your fingers getting numb from the cold, swing your arms around in a circle like a windmill for a few minutes. Windmilling increases blood flow to the hands and fingers, and may delay loss of finger coordination and—in extreme cases—the onset of frostbite.

Frostnip

Frostnip (also called superficial frostbite) is an early cold injury to the skin and does not usually lead to permanent damage. It may progress to deeper frostbite if left untreated.

Signs and Symptoms

Frostnip is usually characterized by numbness of the involved area. Common locations are the fingers, toes, nose, and earlobes. The affected parts will initially appear red and then turn pale or whitish. Frostnipped parts are still soft and pliable to the touch.

Treatment

1. Frostnipped areas should be rewarmed immediately to prevent the progression to frostbite. Place your fingers in your own armpit or groin, and leave them there until they are warm and no longer numb. Place your bare feet on the warm stomach of a companion.
2. Chemical heat packs are also beneficial, but take care not to burn the skin.

Frostbite

Frostbite is freezing of the skin and usually indicates that some degree of permanent damage has occurred.

Signs and Symptoms

Frostbite is recognized by skin that is white and waxy in appearance. The frostbitten part feels hard, like a piece of wood.

Treatment

The best treatment for frostbite is rapid rewarming in warm water as soon as the person can be maintained in a warm environment. Rapid rewarming is preferable to slow rewarming because the damage to tissue occurs during the actual freezing and thawing phases. If possible, avoid rewarming the frostbitten area if there is any danger of refreezing. Walking on frozen feet to shelter is much less damaging than walking on feet that have been thawed. Allowing the feet to refreeze again after thawing is the worst possible scenario.

1. Rapidly rewarm frozen extremities in water at a temperature of 40–41°C (104–106°F). Circulate the water to keep the involved part in contact with the warmest water, and avoid rubbing or massaging the skin. Keep checking the water temperature, as it will cool quickly. Add more hot water if needed. Remove the extremity from the water before adding more hot water.

   Thawing in warm water usually requires 30 to 45 minutes of immersion and can be very painful. Give pain medication before beginning. Thawing is complete when the pale skin has turned to a pink or red color and the skin is soft.

2. After thawing, the involved part will be very susceptible to further injury and should be protected. Application of aloe vera gel to the skin is beneficial in promoting healing of frostbitten skin.
3. When frostbite is rewarmed, fluid-filled blisters (blebs) may form. If this occurs, remove the loose skin overlying the blister and apply aloe vera or antiseptic ointment.
4. Place small sterile gauze pads between toes or fingers, cover the injury with a nonadherent sterile dressing, and loosely wrap the extremity with a bulky bandage.
5. Administer ibuprofen (Advil, Motrin) 600 to 800 mg every 12 hours. Ibuprofen will help relieve pain and may minimize tissue loss.
6. Elevate and splint the affected part.

The depth and degree of the frozen tissue cannot be readily determined by looking at the body part. Even terrible-looking limbs often recover if treated well, so reassure the person and seek professional medical care as soon as possible.

Things Not to Do for Frostbite

1. Do not rub the affected part with snow. In fact, do not massage, rub, or touch the frozen part at all.
2. Be careful not to use water that is hotter than 41°C (106°F), because a burn injury may result.
3. Do not use any form of tobacco. (Nicotine markedly reduces blood flow to the fingers and toes.)
4. Do not thaw the frozen extremity in front of a fire or stove.
5. Do not let the thawed extremity refreeze.
6. Do not walk on frostbitten feet or use frostbitten fingers if possible. (Doing so will cause further injury.)

Immersion Foot (Trench Foot)

Immersion foot, or trench foot, results from exposure to nonfreezing cold and wet conditions over a number of days, leading to damage of blood vessels, nerves, skin, and sometimes muscle, without complete freezing of tissues. In cold environments, sailors, paddlers, and white-water rafters are susceptible to this problem. Trench foot may occur in water as warm as 10°C (50°F) over a 12-hour period, although longer exposure to cold damp environments is the general rule.

Prevention
Boaters should carefully dry and massage their feet and put on dry socks every day, or more frequently. Avoid tight boots, and wear water-proof boots when boating in cold weather.

Signs and Symptoms
- In the early phase, the skin appears blanched and yellow-white in color (waxy). It feels cold to an examiner and to the individual suffering. The foot feels numb or like pins and needles. The sensation is often described as walking on wooden limbs. Balance is impaired, which leads to a shuffling gait.
- During the next few days, the feet become very red and swollen, and then mottled with dark red to blue splotches.
- After rewarming, the feet become hot, painful, red, dry, and swollen. The pain is described as a deep, throbbing, burning ache. Shooting or stabbing pains appear 7 to 10 days later. Subjects cannot tolerate even light pressure on their feet, and bedsheets must be supported on a cradle. In severe cases, large blisters, massive bleeding, and gangrene may appear. Loss of sensation and motor control indicate nerve damage. Blood-vessel injury makes the limb pale when elevated, and bluish-purple when lowered.
- The injury may leave the person with permanent damage and swollen, painful feet, which are extremely sensitive to cold. Muscle wasting may produce weakness and lifelong gait abnormalities.

Treatment
Keep the feet dry and warm, and treat as you would for frostbite, with the exception that rapid rewarming (thawing) is not necessary. Administer strong pain medication as needed. Anti-inflammatory drugs (e.g., ibuprofen [Advil, Motrin]) are not helpful for this condition.

Chilblains

Chilblains can occur in moderately cold, damp climates after repeated exposure to nonfreezing cold and wet environments. Water sports predispose to this type of injury. Sensitivity to pressure caused by footwear is a common complaint.

Prevention

Warm clothing and warm shelter reduce the risk of chilblains. Good foot hygiene, dry feet, and foot massage to stimulate blood flow all help to reduce injury.

Signs and Symptoms

The repetitive cooling of the skin causes spasm and inflammation of the blood vessels, which leads to small localized areas that become swollen, tender, bluish-purple, and itchy. In some cases, blisters just beneath the skin surface develop, and in severe cases, ulceration occurs. Usually, there is no deep-tissue damage, as seen with frostbite or trench foot. Lesions are found on the hands, ears, lower legs, and feet.

Treatment

Treatment modalities for chilblains are similar to trench foot. Topical cortisone cream and drugs that dilate the small blood vessels (e.g., nifedipine [Procardia and others]) may help.

Hypothermia

Hypothermia is an abnormally low body temperature due to exposure to a cold environment. Core (inner body) temperature down to 32°C (90°F) is considered mild to moderate hypothermia, while temperatures below this indicate profound (sometimes called severe) hypothermia. When the body's temperature falls below 28°C (83°F), the heart becomes irritable and is prone to lethal irregular heart rhythms, such as ventricular fibrillation. Death from hypothermia is likely to occur at around 24–27°C (75–80°F). Although few people freeze to death in the backcountry or aboard small boats, the side effects of even mild hypothermia, such as poor judgment and incoordination, can have fatal consequences.

How to Recognize and Treat Hypothermia

Hypothermia is often divided into mild and profound cases, based on a person's temperature and behavior. The distinction is important because the treatment and the worry factor are different. It can be hard to tell where one level starts and the other stops without a special low-reading thermometer. Certain signs and symptoms can often be used to gauge a person's level of hypothermia.

Prevention

- For cold-water divers and those who become routinely cold during and after diving, a dry suit with varying layers of insulating undergarments offers the best thermal protection. The ideal dry suit fabric has breathability (permits water vapor from the skin to pass through freely) and resists penetration by external water. Gore-Tex is one such fabric. It should be rinsed in fresh water periodically to remove residual salt, which reduces breathability. Be sure the collar and wrist gaskets of a dry suit provide watertight seals. Sailors should replace leaky foul-weather gear and avoid wearing cotton, which retains moisture and dries slowly.

- Wind-driven evaporation of water on the outside of a dive wet suit is a powerful cooling force even in a warm environment. Wear a Windbreaker over the wet suit during the surface interval, or remove the wet suit and dry off. Remember: peel off, dry off, cover up!

- Polar fleece (a polyester fabric) is a sailor's best friend; it is warm, lightweight, breathes well, and dries quickly even if soaked by saltwater. Wool is the oldest and one of the best insulating materials for cold-weather clothing. Its major disadvantage is its greater weight compared to pile or fleece. Wool is one of the few materials that maintain insulating properties while wet.

- Blood vessels in the scalp do not constrict (shut down) the way the skin vessels do when exposed to cold, thereby allowing heat loss from an exposed head. Wear snug insulating caps made of wool or polypropylene. Balaclavas, which cover the head, neck, and lower face, are desirable for severe conditions. Hoods on foul-weather jackets usually do not fit snugly enough to provide similar protection; however, a combination of cap and hood works well. Divers should add a neoprene hood while diving in cold water and consider wearing a neoprene "beanie" (which fits like a bathing cap) in the tropics. Paddlers can also wear hats or beanies under their helmets to reduce heat loss.

■ The neck also carries a large volume of blood in vessels that are close to the surface and through which large quantities of heat can be lost. A scarf can limit such loss. Neck gaiters have largely replaced scarves and are very effective.

■ The thermal insulation of a diver's neoprene wet suit depends on the tiny bubbles scattered throughout the neoprene. The neoprene itself is only the matrix that supports the bubbles. Thermal protection decreases as the suit (and bubbles) become compressed at increasing depth; in very cold water, therefore, remain at shallower depths where the insulating neoprene is most effective.

■ For hands, mittens are much warmer than gloves.

■ Stay well-hydrated and well-fed during prolonged exposure to the cold, and plan to consume more calories.

■ Provide calories, fluid, shelter, insulation, and dry clothing to anyone who feels cold before hypothermia sets in.

Getting the Most from a Wet Suit

Depending on the quality and how it is used, a wet suit can last 1 to 5 years. A suit may look fine, but if it stops keeping you warm, it needs to be replaced. Shorty wet suits offer little protection from the cold. Heat is lost from the leg muscles while swimming, and legs constitute a larger portion of the exposed skin surface than the torso does. Protect legs (and oneself) from heat loss with a full wet suit. Leaking, torn wet suits allow warm water to exit and cold water to enter with every movement, creating another large heat drain. A wet suit collar is never a tight seal against the neck, and only a hood with a yoke will create an efficient seal.

How We Conserve and Lose Heat

The body's initial response to cold is to conserve heat by diverting warm blood flowing through the skin and muscles (especially the extremities) to the inner vital organs. The skin becomes an insulating layer and less heat is lost to the environment.

Heat is lost through any of four processes:

■ *Radiation*: This is the direct loss of heat from a warm body to a cooler environment. The head and neck account for more than 50 percent of the body's heat loss. Protective clothing, including a hat and scarf or neck gaiter, will help prevent this heat loss.

■ *Conduction:* This is heat loss through direct physical contact between the body and a cooler surface. Rapid and significant heat loss occurs this way after immersion in cold water. Insulating layers of clothing under a dry suit or a thick neoprene wet suit slow the transfer of body heat to cold water. Insulating someone lying on any surface will help prevent this type of heat loss.

■ *Convection:* This is heat loss by air movement circulating around the body and depends on the velocity of wind (windchill factor). Windproof clothing and shelter will help reduce this type of heat loss. In a survival situation, wrapping a garbage bag around one-self, or even using a pack or sail bag as a bivy sack, can help protect from windchill.

■ *Evaporation:* When sweat or water evaporates or dries on the skin or clothing, it cools. Using a vapor-barrier liner under clothing can minimize this type of heat loss. Less recognized is the cooling effect of evaporation from breathing. This can be reduced by breathing through a scarf or face mask. Paddlers wearing wet suits and sailors exposed to wind and sea spray lose heat in this way. Divers cool down during the surface interval between dives as the wind dries their wet suit.

Mild Hypothermia

At 35°C (95°F), a person enters the zone of mild hypothermia.

Signs and Symptoms

■ Sustained, uncontrollable shivering is one of the most reliable early signs of hypothermia. The person feels cold, and shivering reaches its maximum level.

Your Body's Thermostat Is in Your Skin

Your perception of whether you are cold or warm depends on your skin temperature and not on your core temperature. You cannot "feel" your core temperature. Even when your core temperature is normal, if your skin is cold, you will feel cold and begin shivering (a reflex to generate additional body heat through muscle activity). Conversely, if your core temperature is low but your skin is warm, you feel warm and do not shiver, despite becoming hypothermic.

If you warm a hypothermic individual's skin (place chemical heat pads on the skin or give them a hot shower), you extinguish the drive to shiver, cause the blood vessels on the skin to dilate, and cause a drop in blood pressure. Shivering is the way the body rewarms itself. Hot showers interrupt this process and may cause shock and cardiovascular collapse. This happened during World War II to many sailors whose ships had been sunk, and to downed pilots who were rescued from the cold North Atlantic; they later collapsed and died when sent to the "hot showers."

- The person maintains a normal level of consciousness and is alert, but may show subtle changes in mental status, including impaired judgment, confusion, and disorientation. Personality changes, such as uncharacteristic irritability and combativeness, may be present. Coordination and manual dexterity are normal or slightly impaired. Using navigational tools, plotting a course on a chart, or adjusting binoculars may be difficult.
- At 34°C (93°F), the person develops apathy, amnesia, and slurred speech.
- As muscles cool, both strength and balance deteriorate. Sailors risk slipping and falling overboard while walking on wet and rolling decks. Paddlers have difficulty executing maneuvers, and divers experience weakness while swimming and reboarding the dive boat.

Treatment

1. Get the person into shelter or belowdecks and insulated from the cold.
2. After drying the skin, replace any wet clothing with multiple layers of dry insulating garments. If dry clothing is not available, provide an extra vapor barrier with added foul-weather gear or a sail bag.

A windproof layer minimizes convective and evaporative heat loss. Put on nitrile gloves from the medical kit to help warm the hands.

3. Give the person warm food and lots of sugar-containing fluids to drink. Providing calories (fuel) with simple carbohydrate (sugar) foods and sweet liquid drinks will provide added fuel for the person's furnace (shivering) to enable self-generation of internal heat. (Shivering is an extremely effective source of heat production; it has been shown to produce rewarming rates five to six times the resting metabolic rate.) Fluids are equally important to treat dehydration, which always accompanies hypothermia. Elevating the core temperature of an average-size individual 1°F requires consuming about 60 kilocalories worth of a hot beverage. Because 1 L (1 quart) of hot soup at 60°C (140°F) provides about 30 kilocalories, a person would have to consume 2 L (2 quarts) to raise the temperature 1°F. Nevertheless, warm beverages are psychologically beneficial, and drinks with sugar, such as hot chocolate, are preferred because of the calories and energy provided.

4. Heat loss may be slowed by wrapping the person in plastic bags or tarps as well as a sleeping bag. Huddling together will reduce heat loss.

5. Resist the urge to use hot water bottles or heat packs; they can turn off the shivering mechanism and, by themselves, add very little heat to the core. Instead, heat the cabin, build a fire outdoors, or bring water to a boil and have the person inhale the steam.

6. A conscious and shivering hypothermic person is capable of self-rewarming and does not require evacuation if these guidelines are followed. Let the person shiver while you provide encouragement and nourishment.

Profound (Severe) Hypothermia
At 32°C (90°F), a person is profoundly hypothermic.

Signs and Symptoms
Note: Exact temperatures may vary in individual cases.

■ The person becomes weak and lethargic and has progressive alteration of mental state and consciousness (combative or irrational behavior, or coma).

- The person is markedly uncoordinated: unable to walk a straight line, heel to toe, without stumbling.
- At 31°C (88°F), the person will stop shivering (because he can no longer rewarm himself).
- At 30°C (86°F), the person's heart pumps less than two-thirds the normal amount of blood. Pulse and respirations will be half of normal.
- At 28°C (83°F), the heart is very irritable and unstable, and prone to developing irregularities, such as ventricular fibrillation. The person is in danger of sudden cardiac arrest. Rough handling of the person increases the potential for this to happen.

Treatment

Initial treatment is aimed at preventing further cooling and at stabilizing the person prior to evacuation. *Once a person progresses to severe hypothermia and stops shivering, he is incapable of rewarming himself and requires hospitalization and professional medical care.*

1. Handle the person gently. Rough handling may cause the person's heart to fail. Keep the person in a horizontal position. People who are hypothermic also suffer from dehydration and low blood pressure, and an upright position decreases circulation to the brain and heart.
2. Place the person in a sleeping bag, or place blankets or clothing underneath and on top of the person. Any heat that you can provide will probably not rewarm the person but will help prevent further cooling. External heat, in the form of chemical hot packs or hot water bottles, should be wrapped in cloth, to avoid skin burns, and applied to the groin, neck, sides of the chest, and armpits.
3. A person with a significantly altered mental state should not be allowed to eat or drink, because of the potential for choking and vomiting.
4. Rewarming is best done in a hospital, because of the potential complications associated with profound hypothermia. Professional assistance is usually needed to evacuate a profoundly hypothermic person.

CAUTION: First-aid management of hypothermic persons should not be based solely on measurements of body temperature, because obtaining an accurate temperature in the field can be difficult. It is only one consideration along with other observations and signs (such as an altered mental state) in guiding decision making about appropriate treatment.

It may be difficult to distinguish between someone who is profoundly hypothermic and someone who is dead. The profoundly hypothermic person may have a pulse and respirations that are barely detectable. Double-check carefully in a hypothermic person, feeling for the carotid pulse for at least a full minute, because the heart rate may be very slow. Place a cold glass surface next to the person's mouth to see if it fogs up.

Hypothermia: When to Perform CPR

If the person is breathing or has any pulse, no matter how slow, do not initiate CPR, which can actually make the heart completely stop pumping. If there is no sign of a pulse or breathing after 1 minute, what to do next depends on your situation.

If you're alone on land or with only one other person, cover and place the person in a protected shelter (tent, sleeping bag, tarp, canoe) with insulation above and below. If you can, go for help with another person, and stay together for safety.

If there are multiple medics and it is safe to stay with the person, begin CPR, while at least two people go for help. Chest compressions should be done at one-half the normal rate for a profoundly hypothermic individual.

If on a boat and the person is recovered in cold water, begin CPR unless submersion is known to have been more than 60 minutes.

Table 3: Body Temperature—Related Findings*

Core Temperature	Characteristics
37.2°C (99°F)	Normal rectal temperature
37°C (98.6°F)	Normal oral temperature
35°C (95°F)	Maximum shivering
34°C (93°F)	Poor judgment; slower movements
33°C (91.5°F)	Clumsy movements; apathy
31°C (88°F)	Shivering stops; stupor; altered level of consciousness
28.3–30°C (83–86°F)	Heart irritable and prone to arrhythmia
26.6°C (80°F)	Cessation of voluntary motion; pupils unreactive to light
22.2–25°C (72–77°F)	Maximum risk of cardiac arrest
* General guidelines only; marked variations may occur.	

ILLNESSES CAUSED BY HEAT

Heat emergencies encompass a spectrum of illnesses, ranging from such minor reactions as muscle cramps to heatstroke, a life-threatening emergency. It is better sometimes to stay in the shade, or camp indoors next to an air conditioner. The potential for developing heat illness is greatest in an environment that is windless, hot, and humid. When the outside temperature exceeds 35°C (95°F), which is our normal skin temperature, we begin to take on heat from the environment. Evaporation of sweat from the body's surface is the only mechanism left to dissipate heat. If the humidity level then exceeds 80 percent, the ability to lose heat (from evaporation) declines dramatically, and the risk of developing heat illness soars. Sweat that merely drips from the skin and is not evaporated only contributes to dehydration without providing any cooling benefit.

Prevention

Dehydration is the most important contributing factor leading to heat illness. Keep yourself and your crew hydrated. Water requirements change dramatically with exercise, sweating, diet, and changes in ambient wind, humidity, and temperature. When you're overheated, the blood vessels near the skin dilate so that more blood can reach the surface and dissipate heat. If you're dehydrated, the blood vessels in the skin will do the opposite and constrict and you will not be able to cool off as readily. More important, dehydration limits the ability of the body to sweat and evaporate heat.

Unfortunately, the body's dehydration sensor is not very sensitive. It waits until we're already 2 to 5 percent dehydrated before sounding the thirst alarm, and then shuts off prematurely after we have replaced only two-thirds of the fluid deficit. The best way to determine dehydration is by the color of urine:

- Clear to pale-yellow urine indicates that sufficient fluids are being consumed.
- Dark yellow or tan-colored urine indicates dehydration.

It really is that simple! (**Note:** Some vitamins and medications can also turn urine a yellow or orange color.)

During exercise, you can easily sweat away 1 to 2 L (1 to 2 quarts) of water per hour. Trying to keep hydrated requires a continual, conscious effort. Everybody should carry a water bottle where it is easily accessible, and should drink at least 0.5 L (1 pint every 20 minutes during a hike. As a general rule, in a hot environment, a person should drink 4 L (1 gallon) of water for every 32 km (20 miles) walked at night and 8 L (2 gallons) for every 32 km (20 miles) walked during the day.

On an average summer day, sailors should consume an absolute minimum of about 2 L (2 quarts) of fluid. 2 L (2 quarts) of water can be easily lost during an hour of vigorous paddling, especially while wearing a nonbreathable paddling jacket.

Constant exposure to wind and sun requires boaters to consume extra fluids to remain well-hydrated. The evaporative loss from the action of sunlight on someone in an open boat in the tropics is about 2.5 L (2.5 pints) per day, and the body is constantly absorbing radiant heat from the sun. Boaters often fail to appreciate both the heat of the day and the drying effects of the warm breeze. Continuous evaporation of sweat removes the visible reminder of fluid loss, and quick-drying fabrics accentuate this invisible evaporative loss. Signs of overheating also may be less obvious as the body absorbs radiant heat from the sun and the breeze cools the skin.

Limited stores and poor taste of a boat's tank water can reduce voluntary fluid intake. Powdered drink mixes, sports drinks, or fresh lemons and limes can counter bad-tasting water. Caffeinated drinks stimulate fluid loss through increased urination. A cold beer may be refreshing; however, alcohol promotes dehydration by increasing urine volume as well, often more than the amount of fluid initially consumed.

Seasick sailors suffer from dehydration because of recurrent nausea and vomiting. Initiate medication and rehydration early in the illness (see "Seasickness," page 203).

Scuba diving, surfboarding, or swimming in cool water causes blood vessels in the skin to constrict in order to conserve body heat. The kidneys respond to this diversion of blood from the skin to the internal organs by forming more urine, further depleting the body of fluid. After swimming or diving in cool water, always drink extra liquids to replace this loss.

The mandatory daily water requirement for a person at rest is about 1.5 L (1.5 quarts). Approximately 0.5 L (1 pint) is lost through the skin by evaporation, 0.5 L (1 pint) is necessary to humidify inspired air in the lungs, and the kidneys utilize 0.5 L (1 pint) to excrete the waste products of metabolism.

In a survival situation (e.g., stranded in the desert or adrift in the tropics on a life raft), stay as cool as possible by limiting activity and sun exposure during the heat of the day. Without water, survival time varies between 1 and 5 days depending on the ability to reduce sweat loss. The minimal daily requirement to ensure survival (but not optimal fitness) is 120 to 240 mL (½ cup to 1 cup) of water daily.

In a survival situation, drinking seawater is counterproductive and dangerous. It increases dehydration and hastens death. With a salt concentration of 3.5 percent, seawater has about four times the concentration of salt that is found in the human body; therefore, it draws precious water out of the body as the kidneys attempt to eliminate the excess salt. Drinking urine is ill-advised, because of its heavy concentration of waste products.

The colder and tastier the beverage, the more likely you will want to drink it. Colder fluids are more easily absorbed from the stomach. Wrap a drink bottle in an article of clothing to help keep it cool, and add a powdered sports-drink mix after disinfecting the water. The body can absorb a carbohydrate-containing beverage up to 30 percent faster than plain water. Diluted sports drinks (half strength) are ideal. Higher carbohydrate concentrations should be avoided, because they can produce stomach cramps and delay absorption. A sports drink with about 8 percent sugar and some salt works well.

Salt lost in sweating can usually be replaced by a normal diet or by adding a small amount of salt to drinking water. The ideal concentration is a 0.1% salt solution, which can be prepared by dissolving 2 10-grain salt tablets or 1.5 g ($\frac{1}{4}$ teaspoon) of table salt in 1 L (1 quart) of water. The salt tablets should be crushed before attempting to dissolve them. Salt tablets should not be swallowed by themselves without food and fluid; they irritate the stomach, produce vomiting, and do not treat the dehydration that is also present.

- Hiking, fishing, and boating are best done in the early morning and late afternoon when the sun is low and the heat less intense.
- Know the side effects of medications:
  1. Antihistamines and anticholinergics found in many medications for colds, seasickness, and allergies decrease the rate of sweating.
  2. Antihypertension drugs, such as beta-blockers, ACE inhibitors, psychiatric drugs, and diuretics, can predispose one to heat illness.
- Adequate time should be allowed for acclimatizing before exercising for prolonged periods in the heat. It takes about 10 days to become acclimatized to a hot environment. During that time, you will need to do about 2 hours of exercise each day. With acclimatization, your body becomes more efficient at cooling itself and you are less likely to suffer heat illness.

- Wear clothing that is lightweight and loose-fitting for ventilation, and light-colored to reflect heat. The new sun-protective clothing helps keep you cool by blocking UV radiation.
- Get plenty of rest: There is a correlation between lack of sleep, fatigue, and heat illness.
- Avoid sunburn and excessive direct sun exposure. Use a Bimini top for the cockpit when cruising in tropical climates, and wear sun-protective clothing, including a broad-brimmed hat.
- Maintain potable water in the boat's water tanks by removing bad taste and smell (see Appendix A, page 294), or carry large jugs of fresh drinking water.
- Take medication to prevent seasickness before departure and at regular intervals thereafter. Treat nausea and vomiting promptly by administering a promethazine (Phenergan) or prochlorperazine (Compazine) suppository 10 to 25 mg or ondansetron (Zofran) tablets.
- Men with an enlarged prostate tend to restrict fluids in order to urinate less frequently. Women may also restrict fluids to avoid going below to the head in rough weather or requesting a special stop on a paddling excursion. The trip leader or captain must be sensitive to these basic needs so that all maintain good hydration and drink freely.
- In hot climates, cool the body and conserve body fluids by periodically wetting the skin. Seawater, lake water, or river water sponged onto the skin, or water-soaked clothing and hats (especially the quick-drying fabrics), serves as artificial sweat and cools as it evaporates. If possible, swim or splash in the water to hasten the cooling process. Water absorbs heat from the body twenty-five times faster than air at the same temperature. Kayakers should remove their helmets while resting during a break. Use ventilated helmets in warm weather. Clothing can reduce the solar heat load from the sun by more than 50 percent, so cover up with lightweight, well-ventilated clothing and a hat.

Treatment for Dehydration with an Enema

If persistent vomiting prevents oral rehydration, administering clear rehydration fluids via an enema is the best alternative, since the large intestine and rectum normally function to absorb fluid. Do not procrastinate—this procedure may be lifesaving.

To administer an enema, fill the enema bag with warm water (body-temperature or slightly warmer) and have the person lie on the left side with knees drawn up. Don gloves, and gently insert the lubricated tip slowly into the rectum 2.5 to 5 cm (1 to 2 inches). Elevate the bag and let the water flow by gravity alone. Repeat, installing about 0.5 L (1 pint) every 1 to 2 hours until urination is normal or the person is able to take fluids orally.

Heat Edema
Swelling of the hands, feet, and ankles is common during the first few days in a hot environment. It is usually self-limited and does not require treatment.

Prickly Heat
This is a heat rash caused by plugged sweat glands in the skin.

Signs and Symptoms
An itchy, red, bumpy rash develops on areas of the skin kept wet from sweating.

Treatment
1. Cool and dry the involved skin and avoid conditions that may induce sweating for a while.
2. Antihistamines such as diphenhydramine (Benadryl) may relieve itching.

Heat Cramps
These are painful muscle spasms or cramps that usually occur in heavily exercised muscles, and often after excessive water intake without added salt.

Signs and Symptoms
Spasms often begin after exertion has ended and a person is resting.

Treatment
Stretching the muscle usually terminates the cramp. For example, extending the leg and pulling the foot upward (or leaning forward against a wall, with feet flat on the ground) can stretch the calf muscle. Rest in a cool environment is advised, and gentle, steady pressure can be applied to the cramped muscle. Don't knead or pound the muscle—this only contributes to the residual soreness.

Further treatment—as well as prevention—consists of drinking plenty of fluids containing small amounts of salt. Salt tablets taken alone are not advised.

Heat Syncope
When a person stands for a long time without moving (e.g., standing on watch at the helm), blood pools in the legs instead of returning to the heart. Standing in a hot environment also causes blood vessels on the surface of the skin to dilate, taking more blood away from the heart, which means less blood is traveling to the brain.

Signs and Symptoms
The combined effect of blood pooling and blood vessels dilating can cause someone to faint from insufficient blood flow to the brain.

Treatment
Lying in a horizontal position with the legs elevated and cooling the skin will treat this condition.

Heat Exhaustion
Heat exhaustion is the most common form of heat illness.

Signs and Symptoms
- Malaise, headache, weakness, and loss of appetite
- Nausea and vomiting (common)

- Dizziness (feeling faint) when standing up from a sitting or lying position
- Dehydration
- Core temperature ranging from normal to moderately elevated (to 40°C [104°F])
- Sweating, normal mental state, and normal coordination

Treatment
1. Stop all exertion and move the person to a cool and shaded environment.
2. Remove restrictive and most other clothing.
3. Administer oral rehydration solutions with plenty of water.
4. Place ice or cold packs alongside the neck and chest wall, under the armpits, and in the groin. Other cooling methods include fanning while splashing the skin with tepid water, or soaking the person in cool water (a stream, bay, lake). Wearing wet clothing in a low-humidity environment will also promote evaporative cooling. Simply dumping a hat full of river water over the head can be very cooling.

   WARNING: Do not place ice directly against the skin for prolonged periods.
5. Physical activity should be resumed only after the person has completely restored body fluids and demonstrates normal urine output and normal urine color.

Heatstroke

The difference between heatstroke and heat exhaustion is that persons with heatstroke have abnormal mental states and abnormal neurological function. They may be confused, or display erratic or bizarre behavior, be disoriented, or seem off-balance (the person may appear intoxicated and unable to walk a straight line). Seizures and coma are late manifestations. Sweating may still be present in heatstroke. Dry, hot skin is a very late finding and may not occur in some persons. Therefore, those who have a temperature above 40°C (105°F) and an altered mental state should be considered to have heatstroke, whether or not they are still sweating.

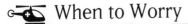 When to Worry

Heatstroke

Heat exhaustion that is not treated can progress to full-blown heatstroke, which is a life-threatening medical emergency. Anyone suffering from heat illness who has an altered mental state (bizarre behavior, confusion), should be treated for heatstroke with rapid cooling, and transported to a hospital.

Signs and Symptoms
- *Best sign:* Altered mental state (confusion, disorientation, bizarre behavior, and delirium)
- *Present or absent:* Sweating
- Elevated temperature, usually above 40°C (105°F)
- Rapid heart rate and respirations
- Low blood pressure
- Stumbling, loss of coordination and balance
- Seizures, coma

Treatment
CAUTION: Do not give the person anything to drink, because of the risk of vomiting and aspiration. (They will later require fluid replacement.) Also, acetaminophen (Tylenol) and aspirin are not helpful in heatstroke and should not be given—aspirin may be harmful.
1. Cool the person immediately and as rapidly as possible. Heatstroke is one of the few true medical emergencies in which a few minutes may significantly alter the outcome. If the person is unconscious, be sure the airway is unobstructed.
2. Place ice or cold packs alongside the scalp, neck, and chest wall, under the armpits, and in the groin, where large vessels come near the surface.
3. Wet the person's skin with tepid water (or any water available, even urine!), and fan the person rapidly to facilitate evaporative cooling.

CAUTION: Do not use alcohol sponging; children can absorb isopropyl alcohol through the skin.

4. During cooling, massage the extremities to help propel cooled blood back into the organs of the body and head. Immerse the person in cool water, if available and if the person is conscious— but always support and hold on to them! Cold-water cooling, even an ice-water bath, is twice as fast and effective as the spray and fan method, as long as it does not cause shivering (which heats the body).

5. Treat for shock (see "Life-Threatening Emergencies II," page 34).

6. Evacuate the person as soon as possible. Continue to cool during the evacuation until the person's rectal temperature falls to 38°C (100–101°F) .

7. Recheck the temperature at least every 30 minutes.

ILLNESSES CAUSED BY SUN

Ultraviolet radiation from the sun (UVA, UVB) causes a variety of health problems for the outdoor and water sports enthusiast. UVB rays are the primary cause of sunburn. Although UVA plays a minor role in ordinary sunburn and tanning, it is responsible for the intense burns and reactions that occur while using medications or cosmetics that make a person more sensitive to the sun (photosensitivity reactions). Both UVA and UVB contribute to the dry, leathery, and wrinkled appearance of the skin (premature aging), skin cancer, and eye damage (cataracts, retinal injury).

UVA levels remain strong all day and all year long. The intensity of UVB varies; it is strongest between 10:00 AM and 3:00 PM, when the midday sun is overhead, and is 400 times more intense in the summer. If you can't see your shadow on a sunny day, or if it's shorter than you are, it's prime sunburn time.

Swimmers and snorkelers can easily burn while in the water, since 80 percent of ultraviolet radiation penetrates 30 cm (12 inches) beneath the surface. Wet skin allows even better ultraviolet penetration and burning. Sunlight is reflected off water, especially from choppy seas. A shade barrier (e.g., hat, boat dodger, or Bimini top) provides incomplete protection for boaters, as harmful rays come from all directions. Reflected rays can burn eyes and undersides of the mouth, nose, and chin. Overcast days afford little relief, since most radiation is transmitted and scattered through the haze and high clouds. Boaters suffer from sunburn often on cloudy days, because they forget to take sun-protective measures.

Sunburn
Prevention

When practical (and it is often impossible), schedule recreational activities on the water in the early morning and late afternoon, when the intensity of UVB is lowest. Sunscreens and clothing offer the best protection against sunburn. Use sunscreens that are rated for UVA and UVB protection; they will be labeled "broad-spectrum." SPF refers only to UVB protection, and not UVA protection. Chemical sunscreens require application 30 to 60 minutes before sun exposure to penetrate and bond to the deep layers of the skin.

Sunblocks (e.g., zinc oxide, titanium dioxide) act as physical shields and reflect or scatter light. These compounds block UVA and UVB completely. They are effective immediately upon application and are ideal for highly exposed small areas, such as the lips, nose, and ears.

Broad-spectrum sunscreens with at least SPF 30 should be applied liberally in amounts according to the label. But how much sunscreen do you need?

"An ounce of prevention" requires an ounce of sunscreen (30 mL)—for one application over the body! This includes 5 mL (1 teaspoon) for the face. Apply it to dry skin 20 minutes before exposure. A sunscreen with SPF 30 blocks 97 percent of UVB, but protection is much less if not applied in a sufficiently thick layer. Many people apply sunscreen unevenly, use insufficient amounts, or fail to reapply it. Reapplication is usually required every 2 hours and after swimming or heavy sweating. Use products that are labeled "water-resistant." (There are no completely waterproof formulas.)

Dry, very tightly knit dark fabrics block almost all ultraviolet radiation. If you want to test the blocking ability of your regular boating clothing, hold it up to a sunny area. If you can see through it, so can the sun. Wearing Lycra suits helps prevent sunburn while snorkeling. While boating, a broad-brimmed hat shades the face, neck, and eyes, adding extra protection. In contrast, a baseball cap does not protect the sides of the face, ears, or neck. Quick-drying, nonstretch fabrics are preferable to cotton (SPF 5–9), which allows 50 percent ultraviolet transmission when wet. People with a history of sun sensitivity, or those who are regularly out in the sun during periods of maximum intensity, should consider purchasing clothing made with special fabrics designed for sun protection. Long pants and long-sleeved shirts are designed lightweight, for comfort, ventilation, and quick drying.

UPF ratings indicate how much UV is blocked by the fabric: 30–49 is very good, 50 or higher is excellent protection. Look for the Skin Cancer Foundation Seal of Recommendation as a reliable standard.

By covering up with clothing, one can avoid the potential adverse health effects of the some of the ingredients in sunscreens. Pregnant women should consult their obstetrician regarding the safety of specific products.

Signs and Symptoms

The redness of the skin that we recognize as sunburn represents underlying inflammation and injury that evolve into first-degree (red) and second-degree (red and blistered skin) burns. The hot, painful burn appears 2 to 6 hours after exposure and reaches maximum intensity a day later. Tissue swelling, blisters, and subsequent peeling often follow.

Treatment

1. Apply cool, wet compresses for 15 to 20 minutes throughout the day; application of cold, wet dressings soaked in a boric acid solution: 5 mL per liter of water (1 teaspoon per quart of water), or a 1:50 solution of aluminum acetate in water, may relieve discomfort.
2. Anesthetic sprays or ointments are effective but can produce significant allergic reactions.
3. Frequent cool showers or dousing the affected areas with cold seawater, lake water, or river water are soothing.
4. Ibuprofen (Advil, Motrin) 400 mg or aspirin 650 mg three to four times a day with food reduces inflammation and controls pain.
5. Topical application of aloe vera gel provides relief and promotes healing.
6. OTC hydrocortisone ointment reduces inflammation and may reduce pain if applied early. However, it may slow healing and repair and may increase susceptibility to infection; use it sparingly.

7. Follow the treatment for second-degree burns (see "Second-Degree Burns," page 142) if blisters are large and extensive.

Photosensitivity Reactions

These reactions are simply exaggerated sunburns or rashes triggered by sun exposure either after taking a particular drug or after coming in contact with a chemical or plant extract. The list of potential offenders is extensive and includes medications, shampoos, perfumes, soaps, lotions, foods, food additives, and even sunscreens (see Appendix B, page 306).

Signs and Symptoms

The sunburn or rash appears immediately and worsens over 2 to 4 days. Some rashes resemble poison ivy with hives.

Treatment

Treat mild reactions as for sunburn. More protracted and severe reactions require oral prednisone (Deltasone and others); the adult dose is 60 mg, reduced by 10 mg daily over the week. A history of no prior reactions does not guarantee safety. Review your medications with your physician, and when possible, substitute drugs with decreased risk of a reaction. If you must take a drug associated with sensitivity reactions, take extra care to protect your skin, and cover up.

Eye Overexposure

Excessive ultraviolet radiation (UV) to the unprotected eye over time can lead to damage of the eye(s).

Signs and Symptoms

Cataract formation (clouding of the lens) and injury to the inner eye (retina) result from excessive UV exposure. A sunburn-like injury (photokeratitis) to the cornea, similar to mountaineer's snow blindness, produces intense eye pain and profuse tearing, with redness, swelling, and spasm of the eyelids. There is a gritty sensation in the eyes, and it hurts to look in bright areas and at lights. The pain and temporary loss of vision start 4 to 12 hours after exposure.

Treatment

Treat by instilling antibiotic ointment or eyedrops, and patching the eyes closed for 24 hours. Administer ibuprofen (Advil, Motrin) and other pain medication as needed. The best protection is wearing a hat with a wide brim, and sunglasses that block both 95 percent UVA and 99 percent UVB, or preferably 100 percent of both (check the labels). Polarized lenses reduce glare. Unless they're specifically treated with UV coating, polarized lenses don't offer UV protection.

Sun Poisoning

Some people experience a severe reaction after intense sun exposure.

Signs and Symptoms

This sickness (not a real poisoning) starts with fever, chills, headache, nausea, and vomiting. Dehydration and collapse may follow because of falling blood pressure.

Treatment

Treatment is similar to that outlined for heat exhaustion (see "Heat Exhaustion," page 227), with the addition of oral prednisone (Deltasone and others) for the most severe reactions. The adult dose is 60 mg, reduced by 10 mg every second day.

Skin Cancer

The rays of the sun (ultraviolet radiation) cause skin cancer. If you notice changes in moles (size, shape, or color), or skin lesions that do not heal, see your physician. Remember the ABCDEs of malignant melanoma, the most serious skin cancer: A for asymmetry (one half is unlike the other); B for border (irregular, scalloped, undefined); C for color (shades of tan, brown, and black, and sometimes red, white, or blue); D for diameter (larger than a pencil eraser); and E for evolving (changing in color, shape, and size over time). Another diagnostic concept is the "ugly duckling sign"—the lesion just looks different from any other skin lesions. Have an annual skin examination by a dermatologist to check for early signs of skin cancer, including malignant melanoma.

LIGHTNING INJURIES

Lightning is a recurrent threat to boaters. Many boats struck by lightning suffer severe damage to electronic systems or are destroyed by fire and explosions. Carrying or wearing metal objects, such as scuba gear, an umbrella, a backpack frame, or even a hairpin, increases the chances of being hit.

To calculate the approximate distance in miles you are from a flash of lightning, count in seconds from the time you see the flash to the time you hear the thunder ("flash to crash"), then divide by five (e.g., a 15-second interval means you're about 5 km (3 miles) away from the lightning). Do not rely on this method for determining when to relax the safety measures, because lightning typically occurs in multiple locations, and just because some strikes are far away does not mean another is not close. Precautions should not be relaxed until thunder cannot be heard for 30 minutes.

With practice, boaters can predict threatening weather by learning to recognize various cloud formations and squall lines.

Preventing Lightning Injury on Land

- When a thunderstorm threatens, seek shelter in a building or inside a vehicle (not a convertible).
- Occupants in tents should stay as far away from the poles and wet clothing as possible.
- Do not stand underneath a tall tree in an open area or on a hilltop.
- Get away from open water.
- Get away from tractors and other metal farm equipment.
- Get off bicycles and golf carts.
- Stay away from wire fences, clotheslines, metal pipes, and other metallic paths, which could carry lightning to you from some distance.
- Avoid standing in small, isolated sheds or other small structures in open areas.
- In a forest, seek shelter in a low area under a thick growth of saplings or small trees. In an open area, go to a low place, such as a ravine or valley.

■ If you are totally in the open, stay far away from single trees to avoid lightning splashes. Drop to your knees and bend forward, putting your hands on your knees. If available, place insulating material (e.g., sleeping pad, life jacket, or rope) between you and the ground. Do not lie flat on the ground.

Preventing Lightning Injury on or near Water

■ Whenever possible, get out of, off, and away from the water.

■ If scuba diving when a thunderstorm hits, get out of the water.

■ Get off the beach if possible.

■ Get off a boat in a marina or at anchor if possible.

■ Remove wet clothing and wet suits. Foul-weather gear over dry clothing is okay.

■ Remove all metal objects, including jewelry and scuba gear.

■ If caught out in a storm on a windsurfing board, lower the sail and mast, and sit down on the board.

■ On a boat, lower radio antennas, fishing rods, and any other tall devices.
   Note: Preventing injury is really crucial; there is no system or device that can prevent a lightning strike on a boat.

■ Remain in the center of the boat's cabin. Avoid the engine room, companionway, navigation station, and toilet.

■ Keep low in a boat if it lacks a cabin.

■ Stay away from the mast, rigging, and wet sails.

■ Avoid contact with all metal, especially items connected to the lightning protection system. Don't create an electrical bridge by holding two metal objects at once, such as the wheel and a spot-light handle.

■ Avoid areas where bridging between two highly charged areas, or sideflashes, may occur, such as the foredeck, between rigging and mast, or the seat between the outboard engine and steering wheel.

■ Avoid contact with electrical, navigation, and radio equipment after unplugging it. A handheld portable VHF radio, cell phone, or satellite phone is safe to use.

■ Know the local weather forecast and be alert for changes to severe weather. Monitor NOAA Weather Radio on your VHF radio (channel

1, 2, or 3). Avoid areas of thunderstorm activity whenever possible.

- Heed the 30/30 rule: continue lightning precautions for 30 minutes after the "flash-to-crash" interval exceeds 30 seconds (10 km [6 miles]).

Types of Lightning Injuries

A common mechanism of injury is for someone to be hit by lightning "splash"; this occurs when a bolt first hits an object, such as the mast or a radio antenna, and then "jumps" to a person nearby.

- *Heart and lung injuries:* Lightning can cause cardiac arrest and paralyze the muscles used in breathing. The heart will often restart on its own, but because the muscles are still not working, the heart will stop again from lack of oxygen (see "Lightning Injuries: Treatment," below).
- *Neurologic injuries:* The person may be knocked unconscious and suffer temporary paralysis, especially in the legs. Seizures, confusion, blindness, deafness, and inability to remember what happened may result.
- *Traumatic injuries:* Bruises, fractures, dislocations, spinal injury, and chest and abdominal injuries from the shock wave may occur. Ruptured eardrums can result in hearing loss.
- *Burns:* Superficial first- or second-degree burns are more common than severe burns after a lightning strike; they form distinctive fernlike patterns on the skin.

Treatment

People struck by lightning are not "charged" and thus pose no hazard to medics.

1. The immediate treatment of persons struck by lightning differs from other situations in which multiple people have been traumatized. Rather than adhere to the standard mass-casualty response protocol of ignoring those people who appear dead and giving priority to those who are still alive, after a lightning strike do the reverse: treat those persons first who appear dead, because they may ultimately recover if quickly given mouth-to-mouth rescue breathing with CPR.

2. If you're successful in obtaining a pulse with CPR, continue rescue breathing (without chest compressions) until the person begins to breathe independently (the breathing muscles will recover) or you are no longer able to continue the resuscitation.
3. Stabilize and splint any fractures.
4. Initiate and maintain spinal precautions if indicated.

CARBON MONOXIDE HAZARDS

Carbon monoxide (CO) is a colorless, odorless, tasteless, and non-irritating gas. In high concentrations, it can be a silent killer in tents and RVs, and aboard houseboats and other sailing and power vessels. The gas binds to the red blood cells and prevents the normal transfer of oxygen and carbon dioxide to and from the tissues during the circulation of blood throughout the body. The result is gradual asphyxiation through insufficient oxygen. The gas is a by-product of combustion of carbon-based fuels such as gasoline, diesel, kerosene, natural gas, propane, coal, charcoal, and wood (not alcohol).

Common sources of CO are main or auxiliary engines, generators, space heaters, cooking stoves, and water heaters. CO can collect from an engine or generator exhaust leak, an improperly vented appliance, or a boat moored or docked too close to another boat that is running a generator or engine. Houseboats that have a generator venting into the enclosed space under the stern swim platform place swimmers at risk in that area. Many children have died from CO exposure while swimming at the stern.

CO is also a hazard for scuba divers, who can become poisoned by breathing contaminated gas from their tanks. CO can enter the tanks during refills, when exhaust fumes enter the air intake of a compressor, or by combustion of lubricants within the compressor itself.

Prevention

- Maintain fresh air circulation throughout the boat or RV at all times.
- Be sure exhaust systems are properly maintained and appliances correctly vented.
- Never hang on the back deck or teak swim platform while the engines of a boat are running. "Teak surfing" is never a safe activity.

- Never enter areas under swim platforms where exhaust outlets are located.
- Run exhaust blowers on a boat whenever the generator is operating.
- Be aware of prevailing wind conditions and back drafts at a dock, a mooring, a seawall, or when motoring downwind.
- Install carbon monoxide detectors in accommodation spaces (at eye level), and make sure the spaces are well-ventilated. Test the alarms regularly.
- Periodically inspect exhaust systems for leaks and for corroded or cracked fittings.
- Listen for changes in exhaust sounds that might indicate a defect or component failure.
- Practice preventive engine maintenance and keep engines tuned.
- Always fill your scuba tank from a reputable dive center that monitors its equipment. (Some monitor the quality of compressed air with electronic CO detectors.)

Signs and Symptoms
The effects of exposure to CO are cumulative.

- Mild symptoms include headache (the most common symptom), burning irritated eyes; drowsiness; fatigue; balance problems; nausea; vomiting; and dizziness. These symptoms mimic seasickness, food poisoning, and flu-like illness, and hence, often lead to misdiagnosis.
- More severe symptoms are difficulty breathing, chest pain, and pounding heart rhythms (palpitations).
- CO affects the brain, leading to difficulties with vision, ringing in the ears, seizures, loss of consciousness, and eventually, coma.
- In some cases, the skin and lips appear "cherry red."
- Almost half of the people with significant CO exposure develop delayed symptoms, arising from 3 to 240 days after apparent recovery. They experience variable degrees of confusion, decreased ability to problem solve, personality changes, loss of balance, and muscle incoordination. These symptoms may persist for a year or longer.

Treatment

1. The most important intervention in the management of CO poisoning is prompt removal of the person from the source of CO into fresh air.
2. Administer pure oxygen by high-flow face mask if available. (Oxygen and mask can often be found on a nearby dive boat.) If oxygen is not available and the symptoms are mild, the person will recover over 4 to 8 hours by simply breathing fresh air.
3. Comatose persons should be evacuated, as should pregnant women and people with heart disease.
4. Rescue breathing may be required.
5. For persons suffering from severe poisoning, a hyperbaric chamber (a decompression chamber for scuba divers) may be used to give a higher dose of oxygen. Use the Divers Alert Network emergency number (1-919-684-9111) to locate the nearest chamber (see "Divers Alert Network," page 248).

DROWNING AND SUBMERSION INJURY

Drowning is defined as death secondary to suffocation while submerged in a liquid, or within 24 hours of submersion. Submersion injury, often called "near drowning," is survival beyond 24 hours after a submersion episode, regardless of the duration or extent of recovery.

Prevention

Drowning accounts for the majority of fatalities in accidents involving open motorboats under 8 m (26 feet), sailboats, white-water rafts, canoes, kayaks, and other small nonmotorized craft. Capsizes and falls overboard are the most common cause of drowning. Alcohol consumption is often a contributing factor. Of the drowned persons found without life jackets, 85 percent of their deaths were preventable had they worn one.

Life jackets really do save lives. Paddlers should wear an appropriately rated and fitted life jacket and know white-water swimming techniques. Nonswimmers and children should always wear a life jacket aboard any recreational boat. Sailors should wear a life jacket and safety harness in rough weather, at night, during conditions of poor visibility, when seasick, during maneuvers where there is a risk of falling overboard (e.g., sail changes, spinnaker takedown), and whenever alone on watch. Crew should practice "Man overboard" recovery procedures. Life jackets should be comfortable, well-fitting, and appropriate for the activity, swimming ability, and size of the individual.

River paddlers face the possibility of drowning after entrapment. Water can travel through undercut rocks or strainers (e.g., fallen trees), trapping swimmers and boats. Scouting rapids and knowledge of hidden hazards in local rivers can reduce the risk. Entrapment can also occur while walking in shallow moving water; if a foot becomes wedged between rocks, it may be impossible to regain one's balance and stand upright against the force of the current.

Rip currents account for the majority of rescues performed by surf beach lifeguards. These powerful channels of water flowing away from shore at surf beaches (even Great Lakes beaches) can quickly sweep a strong swimmer out to sea. Rip currents typically form at breaks in sandbars and near coastal structures, such as jetties and piers. Visible clues that a rip current is present are a channel of churning, choppy water; a break in the incoming wave pattern; a difference in water color; and a line of foam, seaweed, or debris moving seaward.

If caught in a rip, stay calm and don't panic or try to fight the current. It will not pull you under, but it will pull you away from shore. To escape, swim in a direction following the shoreline, and when free of the current, continue to swim away from it at an angle toward shore. If unable to swim out of the rip, tread water or float until it weakens (which it will), and then swim out of it.

Of prime importance in submersion incidents is the safety of the medics. Whenever possible, throw a life ring or other flotation device to someone who is struggling. Rescues from the beach are best accomplished with a surfboard or other sturdy flotation device.

Scuba divers can decrease their risk of drowning by following some basic principles:

- Don't drink alcohol immediately before diving.
- Always dive with a buddy. Your buddy can provide assistance in case of injury, entanglement, equipment problems, or running out of air. If you expect to be briefly away from each other, use a dive float and flag to identify your location.

- Watch your pressure gauge, and plan to surface with at least 500 psi in reserve. Consider carrying an emergency alternative air source such as Spare Air, which provides enough air to safely return to the surface.
- Develop prudent and conservative diving habits and dive well within the established limits of the dive tables (they're based on healthy young Navy divers).
- Maintain good health and fitness.
- Inform the dive master of medications taken and of existing medical conditions that might become problematic (e.g., diabetes, asthma) during or after a dive.
- Practice quick release of a weight belt or weights integral to the buoyancy vest.
- The surface can be especially hazardous in choppy seas. Put air in the buoyancy vest for ample flotation on the surface, and keep your back to the waves to protect your mouth and nose.
- Know your limits for diving, obtain refresher courses periodically, and remember that even if you do everything right, there is still an inherent risk.
- Whatever the emergency while diving, try to stay calm and confident, and do not panic.

What Does Drowning Look Like?

Drowning is almost always a deceptively quiet event, especially for children. It is not the waving, splashing, and yelling for help that most people expect but rarely see. Of the approximately *750 children* who drown each year, about *375 of them* will do so within 23 m (25 yards) of a parent or other adult. *In 10 percent of those drownings, the adult will actually watch them drown, having no idea it is happening* (source: Centers for Disease Control and Prevention). Drowning does not look like drowning. Respiration takes priority over calling for help in the brief moment the mouth is above the water surface; the mouths of drowning people are not above the surface of the water long enough for them to exhale, inhale, and call out for help. Drowning people press their arms down on the water surface to lift their mouths out of the water to breathe—they cannot perform voluntary arm movements such as waving for help or reaching for a piece of rescue equipment. They remain in a vertical upright position and struggle on the surface of the water from 20 to 60 seconds before submersion occurs.

Look for these other signs of drowning:
- Head low in the water, mouth at water level
- Head tilted back with mouth open
- Eyes glassy and empty, unable to focus
- Eyes closed
- Hair over forehead or eyes
- Not using legs—vertical
- Breathing rapidly or gasping for air
- Trying to swim in a particular direction but not making headway
- Trying to roll over on the back

Treatment

1. If a drowning person is not breathing, mouth-to-mouth rescue breathing is the most important first-aid treatment that will increase the person's chance of survival (see "Rescue Breathing," page 27). Use immediate and aggressive measures if trained to do so, even while the person is in shallow water. Once ashore, do not perform a Heimlich maneuver unless you are unable to breathe air into the person because of an obstructed airway. A Heimlich maneuver does not drain water from the lungs and will produce vomiting and aspiration.
2. Expect the person to vomit during rescue breathing; most do. Logroll the person sideways and sweep out the vomitus from the mouth as needed.
3. Note evidence of trauma and undertake spine immobilization if indicated by the mechanism of the event (e.g., diving into a rocky area, swimming a big rapid; see "Spinal Injury," page 94).
4. Check for a pulse and begin chest compressions if necessary.
5. Remove wet clothing and cover the person with blankets or other dry, warm material to prevent hypothermia. Be sure to prevent conductive heat loss by also placing material between the person and the ground or other cold surface.
6. Anyone who has been submerged, including those who spontaneously recover without rescue breathing, require evaluation and observation at a medical facility.

7. Lung injury from inhaled water may develop within minutes, or slowly over 24 hours. The person may appear fully recovered but may later develop respiratory distress. Early signs of lung inflammation from inhaled water and the resulting low blood oxygen level are shortness of breath, agitation, coughing, burning in the chest, and a rising pulse and breathing rate.

8. Administration of oxygen (often available on a dive boat) and inhalation of the bronchodilator albuterol can help ease labored breathing while awaiting evacuation.

9. Without hospitalization and advanced life support, the survival chances are near zero for any drowning person in cardiac arrest. CPR should never be instituted if the boat and crew are placed in grave danger.

10. Following a witnessed drowning in warm water (temperature higher than 10–15.5°C [50–60°F]), discontinue CPR if there is no pulse after 30 minutes, since there is virtually no chance of survival with ongoing CPR.

Following drowning in cold water (temperature lower than 10–15.5°C [50–60°F]), several persons have been revived even after 20 minutes of submersion (and a few have survived after more than 60 minutes). These remarkable saves are presumably due to the protective effects of profound hypothermia on the heart and the brain, effects that may provide a chance for recovery.

If possible, perform CPR on cold-water drowning persons until they reach the hospital or until help arrives. If the pulse does not return within 30 minutes, and evacuation is not imminent, discontinue CPR. In cold-water submersion, do not begin CPR if there is an obvious lethal injury, if the person is frozen (e.g., ice formation in the airway or in the mouth), or if the person is known to have been submerged for more than 60 minutes.

Cold-Water Immersion

Sudden immersion in cold water (temperature lower than 10–15.5°C [60°F]) initiates a series of reflexes that increase the risk of drowning even for the best swimmers. It is suspected that almost half of the worldwide 140,000 deaths happen annually in open water—especially those resulting from sudden immersion in cold water—are due not to hypothermia but to the physiological responses that occur within the first minutes of immersion. Rapid cooling raises blood pressure, heart rate, and the workload of the heart, making it more susceptible to dangerous and life-threatening rhythms. Upon sudden cold-water immersion, an immediate gasp occurs, followed by rapid and deeper breathing. These responses can quickly lead to accidental inhalation of water and drowning.

If you fall into cold water, make a conscious to effort bring your breathing under control immediately. Remain calm, don't panic, and slow your breathing. Swimmers can experience difficulty synchronizing their swim stroke with these changes in breathing and can easily drown, even in calm waters. Better to tread water and get your breathing under control.

Breath-holding time is reduced in sudden cold-water immersion, making escape from a capsized vessel more difficult; kayakers and canoeists have less time to set up and roll their craft upright. When the muscles and nerves in the extremities cool (over a period of about 30 minutes in very cold or icy water), swimming becomes arduous and ineffective. Don't expect to swim a distance that you could swim under more normal conditions. Loss of muscle strength makes it difficult to perform basic survival procedures. Sailors who fall overboard become incapacitated and are often too weak to climb back into a boat, climb the ladder of a rescue craft, or simply grasp a rescue line. Persons in cold water quickly lose the ability to rescue themselves or even assist in their own rescue.

If you fall into cold water, be prepared for violent shivering and intense pain. Remember the sequence and approximate duration of events after sudden unplanned immersion in frigid (icy) water as "1-10-1":

- 1 minute of gasping, when you need to control your breathing
- 10 minutes of meaningful strength to pull yourself out of the water
- 1 hour before you lose consciousness

You can help slow the rate of cooling, and possibly double your survival time, by adhering to the following guidelines.

Guidelines for Survival

- Keep your clothing on while awaiting rescue. Clothing traps air, which provides insulation and buoyancy; trapped water next to the skin is warmed, retarding further heat loss. This is similar to the protective effect of a diver's wet suit. While keeping you warm, the added weight of clothing and boots will not impair your ability to float. If a short swim is your best chance of survival, only then should you remove any extra clothing and footwear.

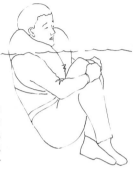

Fig. 73
Heat Escape Lessening Posture (HELP)

- If wearing a life jacket, assume the Heat Escape Lessening Posture (HELP) (**Fig. 73**). Cross your hands over your chest and press your arms closely to your sides; draw your knees up toward your chest and cross your ankles.

- If possible, cover your head and neck, where 50 percent of the heat loss occurs; try to keep your head above water at all times.

- If you don't have a life jacket, move slowly and tread water using slight movements. Exercise wastes precious energy and accelerates the rate of cooling by increasing blood flow to the extremities. Activity also flushes cold water through clothing, increasing heat loss.

- Avoid long swims. Swimming is an option only if likelihood of rescue is low. A fit swimmer wearing a personal flotation device (PFD) might be able to swim 0.6 km (0.4 mile) in 10°C (50°F) water before loss of muscle strength. Pace yourself with an easy stroke that keeps your head and face out of the water (e.g., the breaststroke).

- Always reboard or climb on top of a swamped or capsized boat and await rescue. Once out of the water, stay out, no matter how cold the air temperature, the windchill, or how chilled you feel. You'll always survive longer out of the water. The body cools faster in water than in air, because the rate of heat transfer from skin to water is 25 times greater than in air at the same temperature.

Survival Tips for Scuba Divers

- Peeing in your wet suit will not make you warmer. Cold skin is a better insulator than warm skin because the blood vessels near the surface constrict and less body heat is lost.
- Wear a suit that fits well—not so loose that it fills with water.
- Wear a hood or a beanie in cold water.
- If you feel cold and begin to shiver, stay shallow. Below 18 m (60 feet) the average wet suit loses more than half its insulating value.
- Sustained shivering indicates it's time to get out.
- Take off your wet suit during the surface interval, dry your skin, and put on warm clothes.
- Tropical (27°C [80°F]) water can also chill you—consider wearing a thin wet suit or top.

Treatment

Persons who avoid drowning still face the risk of acute hypothermia as the body's core temperature decreases.

1. If the person is fully awake and shivering, then treatment for mild hypothermia (see "Mild Hypothermia," page 216) is reliably effective and evacuation is unnecessary. A person is capable of generating internal rewarming heat by sustained vigorous shivering if given fluids and carbohydrates, but fuel is required for continued shivering.

2. If dry, insulating clothing is not available, provide an extra windproof vapor barrier by dressing the person in foul-weather gear to minimize heat loss.

3. When practical, wrap the person like a burrito in blankets, sleeping bag, sails, or sail bag.

4. After prolonged cold-water immersion, generally more than 2 hours, it is prudent to evacuate the person to a medical facility. Such persons are perilously close to losing both consciousness and the shivering reflex. They are incapable of rewarming themselves, and they require more aggressive and sophisticated rewarming methods.

5. Careful monitoring is required because of the many metabolic complications arising from advanced hypothermia. Some sailors

have been rescued at sea after prolonged cold-water immersion in an apparently stable and conscious state, only to collapse later while walking around the rescue craft or while taking a hot shower. These people are near severe hypothermia and have low blood pressure. Their condition will rapidly deteriorate with activity and during any attempt at external rewarming. They must be kept still, in a supine position, and handled gently in order to avoid physically stimulating the heart to change its rhythm or stop beating.

6. During helicopter evacuation, use a litter with straps so the person can remain horizontal and securely bundled. The rotor blades create a windchill from the downwash and can increase the level of hypothermia. Dress and wrap the person properly during transfer.

The Divers Alert Network

The Divers Alert Network (DAN) in Durham, North Carolina, is available 24 hours a day to assist in the evaluation and initial treatment of diving accidents and provide a referral to the nearest recompression facility.

Emergency hotline: 1-919-684-9111

BAROTRAUMA: INJURIES OF DESCENT

Enclosed air-filled spaces in a diver's body, such as the middle ears, sinuses, and lungs, become smaller in volume as water pressure increases with descent, and expand back to their normal volume with ascent. These spaces require equalization to the pressure at different water depths, or serious damage, known as barotrauma, may result. Such disorders typically occur close to the surface, where the relative pressure changes most rapidly—approximately 25 percent in the first 2.5 m (8 feet), and another 20 percent (nearly a total of 50 percent) in the next 2.5 m (8 feet). At a depth of 10 m (33 feet) or 1 atmosphere the pressure has increased 100 percent, but descending from 10 to 30.5 m (33 to 100 feet) only increases the pressure another 100 percent. No wonder divers have to equalize the pressure in their ears so frequently early in the descent. Upon descent, the injury, commonly referred to as a squeeze, occurs as tissues engorged with fluid and blood are pulled inward in an attempt to equalize pressures.

Prevention

To prevent a squeeze injury, pressurization (inflation) of the middle ears and sinuses should begin on the surface prior to descent (some divers begin a few hours before the dive). Gentle inflation should be repeated every 0.5 m (2 feet) for the first 3.5 to 4.5 m (10 to 15 feet), then often enough to maintain a positive pressure in the middle ears. At a minimum, "strive at five": try to clear your ears every 5 feet (1.5 m). If you have difficulty doing so, ascend 1.5 m (5 feet) to relieve the pressure and try again. At the first sign of discomfort, stop and ascend until symptoms clear, then equalize, and attempt descent again.

Descending feetfirst is better for ear clearing. If possible, control the rate of descent with an anchor line or descent line. Look up and extend your neck (look upward to the sea surface), which helps open the eustachian tubes.

Judicious use of oral decongestants and nasal sprays is acceptable prior to diving to reduce temporary and minor congestion in the nasal and ear passages. Take medication at least 1 hour prior to descent. When cold or allergy symptoms are severe, it is wise to avoid diving until the symptoms resolve. Earplugs and tight-fitting hoods should never be used while diving, because they create air spaces in the external ear canal that cannot be equalized. Avoid the buildup of wax in the external canal, which may also create an air space in the external canal.

Ear Squeeze

The eustachian tube provides a vent that normally equalizes the pressure across the eardrum. It is situated between the middle ear and the throat. If a diver cannot continuously equalize the pressure in the middle ear by gently forcing air through the eustachian tube, gently exhaling (blowing) through the nose while closing the mouth and pinching the nostrils, or by swallowing or yawning, may help. Remember to equalize early, often, and gently.

Signs and Symptoms

If equalization fails, as little as 0.75 m (2.5 feet) of descent below the surface can produce enough pressure to cause ear pain. At 1.2 m (4 feet), the eustachian tube collapses and equalization is nearly impossible. Rupture of the membrane can occur between 1.5 and 5 m (5 and 17 feet). A rupture allows water to enter the middle ear, causing ear, jaw, or neck pain (rarely, no pain); nausea; vomiting; dizziness with loss of balance; disorientation; a ringing or roaring sound in the ear; and hearing difficulty. Milder injuries produce a sensation of fullness, ear pain, and dizziness. If one attempts to forcefully equalize the middle ear pressure once the eustachian tube is blocked, pressure can be exerted on the middle ear from the inner ear, which can then rupture. Such rupture produces more severe disequilibrium and can result in permanent disability.

Treatment

If ear squeeze occurs, the diver must control the feeling of panic and slowly ascend to the surface. Treatment includes decongestants (pseudoephedrine [Sudafed]) and oral antibiotics (the same as for the treatment of otitis). Do not instill eardrops in the event that a perforation has occurred. Persisting symptoms may indicate a nonhealing perforation or more extensive injury involving inner ear barotrauma. If the symptoms are severe, place the diver on bed rest, with the head elevated; avoid coughing, constipation, and any straining with forceful breath holding.

Sinus Squeeze

Sinus squeeze occurs when the openings into the sinuses from the nasal passages are blocked by congestion from infection, inflammation, or allergy. If air cannot enter the sinuses during descent, the lining tissues collapse inward, causing pain and bleeding. The pain is commonly over the eyes or cheeks and is often followed by blood draining into the nose. Slow ascent and treatment with decongestants and antibiotics (the same as for sinusitis) are indicated.

Mask Squeeze

Mask squeeze is a form of barotrauma that occurs when the air cavity within a face mask compresses during descent. Divers experience a pulling sensation on the face and eyes. The surface blood vessels enlarge and may rupture; the eyes appear bloodshot and puffy. The pressure can be equalized by simply exhaling into the mask through the nose. This may cause the mask lens to fog.

Many mask-defogging chemicals cause stinging and eye irritation; a cheap, effective alternative to these chemicals is Crest Cool Mint Gel toothpaste. Just rub it on the mask lens, then rinse it off.

BAROTRAUMA: INJURIES OF ASCENT
Structural Injury
If air enters the chest cavity, the lung may collapse (pneumothorax). Symptoms include shortness of breath and chest pain, which is often sharp and worse with inspiration. Breathing is rapid and shallow, and the diver may appear cyanotic, with bluish lips and fingernail beds. The lung may require insertion of a chest tube to reexpand it; therefore, evacuation to a medical facility is necessary (see "Collapsed Lung [Pneumothorax]," page 65 and "Tension Pneumothorax," page 65).

Air escaping from the lung may also exit to the center of the chest, travel under the skin, and localize around the neck. Signs include changing voice quality, with swelling in the neck and a crackling sensation when the skin is pressed. This in itself is not an emergency, and treatment is not required. However, the diver should be observed for other signs of injury and evaluated for air embolism (see "Air Embolism," page 252).

Reverse Block: Sinuses and Ears
Pain and hemorrhage can also occur in the sinuses when the air expands and is unable to exit the sinus during ascent. This reverse block, or reverse squeeze, is caused by congested openings producing a one-way valve effect. Rarely, there is unequal release of air from the middle ear cavities during ascent, resulting in a pressure difference between the two ears. The diver may experience transient dizziness and nausea, which resolves on further ascent as the eustachian tube opens and allows air to escape.

Lung Overpressurization
The most severe and life-threatening barotrauma involves the lungs. Scuba divers automatically equalize the air pressure in the lungs to the ambient water pressure at depth so long as they breathe continuously

through the regulator, which delivers air at a pressure equal to the surrounding water pressure. Injury occurs during ascent if the expanding gas is prevented from escaping. This commonly occurs with breath holding during a panicked ascent, or by ascending too rapidly without adequately exhaling. Other causes are related to trapping of gas from conditions such as asthma or bronchitis. The expanding air can overinflate, burst a section of lung, and then enter adjacent tissues or spaces in the chest, creating extensive structural injury. Expanding air can also tear the blood vessels in the lung and enter the circulation as gas bubbles. This serious and life-threatening complication is called air embolism (see "Air Embolism," below).

Air Embolism

In cases of air embolism, also called arterial gas embolism (AGE), air bubbles in the circulation may block the blood flow by lodging in the smaller arteries of vital organs, such as the brain or heart, producing a stroke or heart attack. Symptoms appear rapidly during ascent or within 10 minutes of surfacing; rarely, they appear after a longer interval following surfacing. Neurological symptoms are most common and reflect the area of the brain injured; they may be mild, such as numbness or tingling of an extremity, or more severe, such as headache, weakness, or paralysis (a stroke). Other signs and symptoms include changes in vision, speech, or hearing, as well as confusion, seizures, stupor, and coma. Severe chest pain may indicate a heart attack, along with difficulty breathing and a sense of impending doom. Gas embolism is a medical emergency requiring early management similar to that for decompression sickness (see "Decompression Sickness [The Bends]," below).

Decompression Sickness (The Bends)

Compressed air in the scuba tank is a mixture of nitrogen (79 percent) and oxygen (21 percent). The standard scuba regulator allows the tank gas to be delivered at an ambient pressure by using the pressure of the water to regulate flow through a series of mechanical levers. When a diver descends, the increased water pressure causes the nitrogen to be absorbed and dissolved into the blood and body tissue fluids. The deeper and longer the dive, the more nitrogen the body absorbs. The nitrogen is slowly eliminated through respiration as the ambient pressure is reduced during and after the diver's return to the surface.

As long as the amount of absorbed nitrogen is kept within certain limits, the body can safely eliminate it. Decompression illness or decompression sickness (DCI/DCS) is caused by the release of excess nitrogen in the form of tiny gas bubbles into the bloodstream and tissues at depth. The tendency for the formation of nitrogen bubbles depends on the depth of the dive, the bottom time, and the rate of ascent. The many risk factors include obesity, increased age, fatigue, cold, dehydration, alcohol consumption, strenuous exertion during and immediately after the dive, exposure to altitude after a dive, flying after diving, diving deeper than 24 m (80 feet), and a history of a previous DCI/DCS incident. Other contributing elements are deep dives, repetitive diving, missed decompression dives, and multiple no-decompression dives.

Prevention

Recreational diving is often defined as diving that allows immediate ascent to the surface without risk, but in fact, there is no such dive. The major fallacy about decompression theory is the idea that decompression programs in tables and computers can absolutely prevent decompression sickness—in fact, they cannot, so always dive conservatively. Divers should never dive the tables and computers to the limit.

Decompression tables are based on algorithms (mathematical programs), which have had very little testing, derived from simplistic mathematical models of uptake and elimination of gases (from body tissues) at increased pressure while diving. No current model includes any consideration for age, level of hydration, gender, degree of exertion, fitness, or environmental variables such as warm- or cold-water dives, diving at increased altitude, or diving in currents. The tables create a false sense of exactitude—what they describe are not lines but, rather, zones in which caution must be exercised. More than half the divers who experience DCI have made dives that do not conflict with the tables or computer models. Many experienced divers build in conservative "fudge factors" for greater safety margins when using tables: they choose one depth deeper and one time interval longer than the actual planned dive.

Always do the deepest dive first, and limit dives to no more than 40 m (130 feet) (the risk increases at depths beyond 24 m [80 feet]). Poor buoyancy control with rapid ascent is a major factor in DCI cases and AGE incidents. Do not put air in your buoyancy compensator (BC) to start the final ascent—instead, kick upward and inhale to get going. Be prepared to vent your BC as you start up. Ascend at a rate of 9 m (30 feet) per minute or slower, and make a safety stop for 3 minutes at a minimum, and preferably, 5 minutes, at 4.5 m (15 feet). Extend your safety stop time if you can, to breathe out the nitrogen and reduce the bubble risk. The final ascent to the surface should also be gradual: no faster than 30 seconds. Be sure you have neutral buoyancy before you leave the safety stop—you should sink when you exhale. Some dive experts, including the National Association of Underwater Instructors (NAUI), now recommend a deep stop for table-based, no-required-decompression dives—a 1-minute stop at half the maximum depth on all dives deeper than 12 m (40 feet). Once this stop is completed, ascend to the traditional 4.5-m (15-foot) safety stop. Avoid heavy work after a dive, and use assistance to pass up heavy gear to the dive boat, such as weights and the BC with tanks.

Surface intervals allow off-gassing of residual nitrogen. It is therefore important to avoid minimum surface intervals and extend them if practical. Divers should remain well-hydrated and warm, to promote blood flow through the lungs and nitrogen exchange through respiration. To reduce the risk of DCI, divers should not fly for 12 hours after a single no-decompression dive, or for 18 hours after multiple no-decompression dives per day or multiday dives. These are minimum preflight suggested surface intervals; for a greater margin of safety, many experts advise no flying within 24 hours after diving. These same recommendations apply to mountain travel following diving.

Signs and Symptoms

Signs and symptoms of DCI/DCS can appear immediately, while in the water, or within 24 hours after surfacing; most appear during the first hour and persist. They may be subtle, mild, or severe, and can occur anywhere in the body depending on the location and amount of bubble formation. Symptoms may be general, such as excessive fatigue, weakness, dizziness, nausea, malaise, itchy skin, or unusual skin sensations. More localized symptoms may include joint or muscle pain, or pain, numbness, and tingling in the extremities (especially the arms) or torso.

Musculoskeletal pain is the classic form of decompression sickness. The deep, aching pain is poorly localized and often progressive. In 95 percent of cases, it occurs within 6 hours of surfacing. Signs are wide ranging: a change in personality or behavior, a blotchy skin rash, paralysis or weakness anywhere in the body, a staggering gait, coughing spasms, sudden collapse, and coma. Because of the wide array of symptoms and signs, DCI should always be suspected when anything unusual appears in a diver after surfacing. Since more than half the cases of DCI in recreational divers are not associated with violation of safe diving rules, do not disregard any symptom, even when the diver "did everything right." When in doubt, call the DAN emergency number (1-919-684-9111) for consultation.

Treatment

Air embolism and DCS require immediate medical management and recompression in a chamber. If CPR is not required, place the diver in the lateral recovery position, which places the person horizontally on the left side, with the head supported at a low angle and the upper leg bent at the knee. Administer pure oxygen through a mask, and monitor the airway to keep it clear, especially if nausea and vomiting occur. Continue oxygen administration even if symptoms completely resolve, because they may recur, and contact the 24-hour diving emergency DAN number (1-919-684-9111). If air evacuation is used, try to have cabin pressure maintained below 244 m (800 feet) or fly at an altitude of less than 305 m (1000 feet). Even if a recompression chamber is more than a day away, head for the nearest one. The window of opportunity for treatment does not close completely for 2 weeks. Although the *U.S. Navy Diving Manual* recommends recompression in the water as a last resort when no facility is nearby, this is extremely risky, and the dangers outweigh the benefits.

Nitrogen Narcosis

Nitrogen has an intoxicating effect similar to alcohol when breathing air at depths approaching 27 m (90 feet). The deeper the dive, the more pronounced this effect (a depth of 27 m [90 feet] is equal to the effect of one martini; add another martini for each 15 m [50 feet] thereafter). All divers are affected to some degree, and individual susceptibility varies widely. Judgment and coordination are impaired, and behavior may be inappropriate. As with intoxication from any other substance, there is a sense of euphoria. Individuals may appear to perform in a perfectly normal fashion but have no memory of events. They may acknowledge commands but not act on them. Mistakes or risky behavior may result.

The false sense of security and tendency to panic that can accompany nitrogen narcosis are contributory factors in many diving accidents. If early symptoms are unrecognized, the diver may become comatose. Controlled ascent to the surface is the treatment until all symptoms clear. Previous ingestion of sedating drugs and alcohol increases the degree of narcosis. Early recognition is critical. Always dive with a buddy and avoid depths greater than 40 m (130 feet).

HAZARDOUS MARINE LIFE: CREATURES THAT STING

Many types of marine life can be hazardous to boaters, swimmers, fishers, and divers. People playing or working around the ocean should be aware of the potential dangers presented by the marine life residing there. One of the best ways to avoid problems associated with hazardous marine life is to become familiar with these creatures and learn how to avoid illness and injury.

Jellyfish

Jellyfish—including the sea anemone, hydroid, Portuguese man-of-war (bluebottle), sea nettle, Irukandji, and box jellyfish (sea wasp)—inflict painful (occasionally life-threatening) stings. Stings occur when skin comes into contact with the tentacles, which contain millions of venomous stinging cells. These tiny harpoonlike structures, called nematocysts, harbor attached venom sacs to sting their prey. Nematocysts are triggered to fire by contact, such as when touched by the skin of an unwary swimmer. Only a small percentage of the billions of nematocysts present are fired initially; the tentacles remain toxic for months after removal from the water, even after being dried on the beach, and should not be handled. Treatment consists of deactivating the venom and preventing additional injection of venom by broken-off tentacles on the skin. The venom from the box jellyfish (from northern Australia) can kill in minutes by causing abnormal heart rhythms and cardiopulmonary collapse.

Signs and Symptoms

Reaction to the nematocysts varies according to the type of jellyfish, the venom's potency, and the amount injected. Symptoms after a sting vary from itching and mild burning of the skin to excruciating pain (like a bee sting or worse). The skin turns red, sometimes with an imprint of the tentacles; welts, blisters, localized bleeding, and ulceration may develop. The area can remain sensitive for a month and may be permanently scarred or discolored. Box jellyfish envenomation can kill a child in 5 to 20 minutes. Signs of more severe reactions include agitation, nausea, vomiting, seizures, difficulty breathing, irregular heartbeat, falling blood pressure, and paralysis. Severe allergic reactions may develop (see "Anaphylactic Shock," page 37), and delayed skin allergies are common. Stings to the eyes can cause pain swelling, burning, tearing, blurred vision, and light sensitivity. Eating certain species can be fatal.

WARNING: Regarding Treatment of Jellyfish Stings

1. When stung on the mouth or experiencing any respiratory tract involvement, nothing should be ingested by mouth. Monitor the person's condition constantly to ensure an unobstructed airway, and transport the person to definitive medical care.
2. If the sting is from the Australian box jellyfish, use only vinegar, *not rubbing alcohol*. (Jugs of vinegar are available along some stretches of public beaches in Australia.) Seek immediate assistance in addition to completing the following steps. An antivenin is available. Use the pressure immobilization technique (see "Pit Viper Envenomation: Treatment," page 198) to delay absorption of venom from the sting site into the body's general circulation.
3. Don't let anybody convince you that urinating on a jellyfish sting is an appropriate treatment. The acidity is wrong, the salt content is low, and there's no ammonia in it. In some cases, urine even may be harmful.

Prevention

- Keep a bottle of vinegar nearby when swimming or diving in waters with jellyfish.
- Wear a thin Lycra dive suit or some form of protective clothing when swimming, diving, or surfing near coral reefs and jellyfish.
- Be aware of surface concentrations of jellyfish, and always check snorkel and regulator mouthpieces for tentacle fragments.
- Do not dive headfirst into infested waters.
- Jellyfish can become entangled on lines in the water. When diving, do not hold onto the anchor line or the descent/ascent line without wearing gloves.
- Hydroids often grow on submerged lines, rocks, pilings, and boat bottoms. Avoid walking on submerged rocks, and wear protective clothing when cleaning fouled boat bottoms.
- Be alert for the blue gas-filled float of the Portuguese man-of-war (float is about 9 cm [3.5 inches] in diameter). Give it a wide berth to avoid the tentacles trailing beneath the float. Scuba divers should look up while ascending.
- Pay attention to warning signs posted on public beaches.
- Lands End Oil Sea Sting Ointment can neutralize the venom of jellyfish, as well as fire coral and sea lice. The active ingredient, ozone, oxidizes the venom and prevents the rash from forming. Safe Sea Jellyfish Sting Protective Lotion contains chemicals that significantly reduce the frequency and severity of stings from some species of jellyfish and fire coral, as well as sea lice bites (see "Sea Lice," page 264). It is also available in combination with sunscreen.

Treatment

1. Immediately apply vinegar (5% acetic acid) to the affected area to inactivate the venom. If vinegar is not available, flush the area with seawater. Do not rinse with fresh water or apply ice directly to the skin, this will activate the stinging cells, worsening the pain and injury. Irrigate eye stings immediately by immersing the face in seawater and repeatedly blinking, then rinse with copious amounts of sterile eyewash (saline) for at least 15 minutes. Never irrigate eyes with alcohol or vinegar.

If vinegar or alcohol is not available, use household ammonia (one-fourth strength), or a paste or powder of baking soda. Another alternative is meat tenderizer; it should remain on children's skin for no more than 10 minutes, 15 minutes for adults.

Do not use solvents such as gasoline and turpentine, and avoid rinsing with other products containing alcohol (e.g., perfume, liquor). When possible, consult local inhabitants, fishers, beach lifeguards, and the surfing community to find which decontaminant works best for the jellyfish species in the area.

2. Continue to apply the vinegar for 30 minutes or until the pain subsides. Rarely, vinegar can discharge nematocysts in some species. Rubbing alcohol (40 to 70%) is also effective. (Do not use either for stings from the larger Portuguese man-of-war species).

3. Cold packs or ice in a plastic bag (watch for leaks and surface condensation) may relieve pain. Should pain increase, stop treatment immediately and wash with seawater.

4. Be careful not to touch the fragments with your bare hands. Wear protective gloves if possible. Remove any embedded particles or tentacle fragments using a Splinter Picker or tweezers. Do not rub or scrub the affected area. It will cause the cells to fire.

5. Apply shaving cream or a baking soda paste. Shave the area using a razor, knife, credit card, seashell, or other sharp-edged object.

6. Reapply the vinegar or alcohol soak for another 15 minutes.

7. Apply a layer of 1% hydrocortisone cream twice a day. Aloe vera gel will also provide relief. Try an oatmeal bath after the decontamination and tentacle removal to relieve residual itching. If the skin reaction is severe and prolonged, resembling a severe reaction to poison ivy, treat with a short course of oral prednisone (Deltasone and others). Start with 60 mg for adults and decrease the dose by 10 mg daily over 6 days. Use a lower dose for children, adjusted for age.

8. Seek medical attention if a large area is affected, if the person is very old or very young, or if there are significant signs of illness (nausea, vomiting, weakness, shortness of breath, chest pain, etc.).

9. Most injuries resolve within 24 to 48 hours. Consult with an eye specialist if symptoms persist. Patching the eye closed and using a topical antibiotic for eyes may be helpful.

WARNING: Regarding Treatment of Man-of-War Stings

Hot fresh water at 45°C (113°F) is now recommended for rinsing off the nematocysts of the Portuguese man-of war, and vinegar is *not* suggested as a topical decontaminant. The remainder of the treatment is as stated for jellyfish stings.

Fire Coral

These venomous creatures sting the unwary swimmer upon physical contact. Apply a topical decontaminant immediately, and follow the steps outlined for jellyfish stings. Shaving the skin is unnecessary. The area may also be cut or scraped by the sharp limestone coral skeleton. These wounds are slow to heal and prone to infection. They should be thoroughly cleaned, explored, debrided, and treated as contaminated wounds (see "Managing Wounds," page 119). Wear gloves, boots, and protective clothing, and practice good buoyancy control while diving to prevent accidental contact. When bodyboarding, surfing, or windsurfing, keep your feet off the reef and wear reef shoes.

HAZARDOUS MARINE LIFE: CREATURES THAT PUNCTURE

Sea Urchins

Sea urchin spines are venomous. Puncture wounds from these animals can cause difficulty in breathing, weakness, or collapse.

Prevention

A Lycra shirt or a wet suit provides a modicum of protection when diving or falling onto a coral reef from a surfboard. Puncture-resistant footwear should be worn when diving or surfing on coral reefs or in areas where sea urchins are common.

Treatment

To deactivate the venom, relieve pain, and clean the area, immerse the wound in nonscalding hot fresh water (43.3–45°C [110–113°F]) for 30 to 90 minutes. Without a thermometer to check water temperature, try immersing the uninjured extremity in the water to be sure it is comfortable. Keep refreshing the bath with hot water to keep it at the maximum comfortable temperature. Repeat the immersions immediately if pain recurs.

Remove any visible spines gently to avoid breaking them, and avoid crushing any fragments left in the skin. Do not vigorously scrub the area. Dye leached from a withdrawn spine can initially stain the skin, but it usually disappears in a day or two. If the purple or black "tattoo" persists for more than 48 hours together with persistence of pain, the spine fragment is probably embedded. Surgical removal is required for these and any spines penetrating into or near a joint, especially in the hand or foot. Leave the superficially embedded spines alone if they appear difficult to remove, and do not crush them. If the wound is deep (through the skin into fat and muscle, or penetrating the hand or foot) or shows any signs of infection, administer antibiotics (see "Managing Wounds," page 119, for appropriate antibiotic selection).

Cone Shells (Snails)

These beautiful and highly venomous snails are found in the Indo-Pacific, and reefs off the coasts of Hawaii, Mexico, and California. A less toxic Atlantic species inhabits Florida waters. To be safe, regard all species as dangerous. The snail has a flexible tube, resembling an elephant trunk, which contains a venom-filled tooth (up to 0.5 cm [.025 inch] long). The tooth is fired like a harpoon into the snail's prey (and human hand), and in some cases can remain lodged in the puncture wound. The tooth can penetrate gloves and fabric. The whole apparatus can extend all the way back to the opposite end of the shell, injecting venom into an unsuspecting collector handling the shell.

Treatment for the highly toxic species is similar to that described for sea snake bites (see "Water Mocassins and Sea Snakes," page 266), using the pressure immobilization technique (see **Fig. 72**, page 199). No antivenin is available. Collectors should wear proper gloves and never carry a live cone inside clothing. Be wary of cone shells washed ashore; the snail inside may be alive.

Stingrays

When a ray is startled, it whips its serrated bonelike tail into the intruder. Most often, the stingray is disturbed by an unwary swimmer accidentally stepping on it. Pieces of skin and spine frequently remain in the wound.

The backward-pointing barbs on the spine make removal difficult and traumatic if the entire spine breaks off. Surgical consultation may be required. Injury from a stingray includes both deep puncture wounds or lacerations and envenomation. Symptoms include intense pain, bleeding, weakness, vomiting, headache, fainting, shortness of breath, paralysis, collapse, and, on occasion, death.

Prevention
To prevent injury in waters with stingrays, wear thick-soled booties or fins, and shuffle your feet when entering the water over sandy or muddy bottoms to frighten them off. Remember, stingray spines can easily penetrate rubber and neoprene shoes.

Treatment
Rinse the wound, preferably with fresh water, then immerse the injured area in nonscalding hot fresh water (43–45°C [110–113°F]) for 30 to 90 minutes. Hot water inactivates some of the injected venom. Repeat immediately if pain recurs. Remove any visible pieces of the stinger(s) or sheath, then scrub the wound with soap and water. Vigorously rinse and irrigate the puncture site with hot water using a syringe and 18-gauge catheter tip. Do not attempt to close the wound because of the high risk of infection. If medical care is more than 12 hours away, administer an antibiotic such as ciprofloxacin (Cipro) or levofloxacin (Levaquin).

Starfish
Immerse the wound and remove the spine(s) as you would for a stingray wound (see "Stingrays," above).

Crown-of-Thorns Starfish
The skin covering the sharp, brittle, 2.5-cm (1-inch) spines secretes mucus that contains venom with multiple toxins. The spines can penetrate neoprene, leather, and the soles of sneakers. Symptoms range from intense pain, which may last several hours, to nausea and vomiting. The puncture site becomes tender, red, and swollen, and bleeds easily. A bluish color appears around the puncture site. People sensitive to the toxin may develop an allergic reaction, and multiple punctures with embedded

spines may result in weakness, nausea, vomiting, low blood pressure, and, rarely, paralysis.

Treatment is the same as for sea urchin wounds (see "Sea Urchins," page 260). Most systemic symptoms disappear after the spines are removed.

Scorpion Fish (Lionfish, Zebra Fish, Turkey Fish, Stonefish) and Catfish

The spines contain venom, and puncture wounds cause immediate pain and tissue injury. Immerse the wound in nonscalding fresh hot water, remove the spine(s), and treat as you would for a stingray wound. (See "Stingrays," page 261.)

Seek immediate medical attention if the person appears delirious, confused, or short of breath, or shows other signs of a severe illness. In Australia and other areas in the Indo-Pacific, a stonefish antivenin is available for severe reactions. Recently, lionfish have been found in Caribbean waters.

Billfish (Marlin, Sailfish, Swordfish, Spearfish)

The bills on these fish are used to slash and stun, and occasionally to skewer, prey. Anglers are injured by this same mechanism when landing these fish. The fish may appear exhausted or dead but suddenly begin thrashing wildly when brought near the boat or onboard.

Never assume a freshly landed billfish is harmless. Let a fighting fish continue to fight a little longer before cautiously hauling it onboard. A puncture wound to the head, chest, or abdomen can penetrate vital organs, causing a fatal injury. In the event of a puncture leave the bill in the wound, and cut or saw it off the fish. Basic life support and evacuation are necessary. Minor wounds should be treated similar to other wounds sustained in the marine environment.

Needlefish

These fish have a narrow tubular body ending in a long, sharp beak that can drive into every part of the human body, much like an ice pick. Most accidents occur at night, when the lights of fishers excite and attract the fish, causing them to jump out of the water and skim the surface at speeds up to 61 km/h (38 miles per hour). Those fishing at night should be aware of this hazard, and scuba divers should submerge before turning on dive lights. The wounds are at high risk for major internal injury or infection, and often contain a broken retained beak. Treat the injury as a stab wound. Removal of the beak, and evaluation of deep tissue and internal injuries, require evacuation to a hospital.

HAZARDOUS MARINE LIFE: CREATURES THAT BITE

Sea Lice

Sea lice are small crustaceans living on the sandy bottom that often bite the hands and feet of swimmers. The sharp bite is painful and leaves pinpoint hemorrhages. Scrub the skin with soap and water or dilute hydrogen peroxide, and apply antibiotic ointment.

Sharks

Approximately 30 out of 350 shark species have been implicated in human attacks. The most dangerous are the great white, tiger shark, bull shark, hammerhead, grey reef, blacktip, spinner, whitetip, and blue. In the United States, great whites are found in Northern California, bull sharks are found from Florida to New Jersey, and tiger sharks cause most of the attacks in Hawaii.

The odds of a shark attack in North America are 1 in 10 million. There are about 100 attacks yearly worldwide, and less than 10 percent are fatal. More shark injuries occur when anglers land a shark and bring it aboard.

The greatest chemical attractant for sharks is fish blood (they can detect 1 part per billion). Human menstrual blood does not appear to create a particularly dangerous situation for women.

Prevention

Divers and anyone spearfishing should be knowledgeable in shark avoidance and repulsion techniques. Leave the water if you are bleeding from an injury, and remove speared fish from the water as soon as possible. If you have an unexpected encounter with a shark, move away slowly, exit the area, and do not create an underwater commotion or splash at the surface, simulating a struggling fish or seal. It is crucial not to imitate a wounded fish or seal by swimming erratically on or near the water surface. Surfers risk attack by swimming on their boards; a surfer's silhouette on the surface resembles a seal or sea lion from below.

If facing a shark, back up against a fixed object to reduce the possible paths of attack. Many sharks attack from below or from the side. Sharks are best driven off with blunt blows to the snout, eyes, or gills, preferably not with a bare hand. It may be reassuring to know that rescuing someone attacked by a shark is reportedly safe, because sharks rarely attack twice.

Treatment

Shark bites cause severe tissue damage; death is usually due to hemorrhage and shock. All bites from marine animals, however minor, are at high risk for infection; the wounds should be thoroughly cleaned using high-pressure irrigation (see "Managing Wounds," page 119), and should not be sutured or taped tightly shut. Allow the wound to drain and begin antibiotic therapy. When feasible, wounds should be explored in the operating room. Skin abrasions from contact with sandpaperlike shark skin should be cleaned with soap and water and covered with antibiotic ointment and a sterile dressing.

Barracudas

Barracudas have two parallel rows of exceptionally sharp cutting teeth in both the upper and lower jaws. They can inflict deep, slashing cuts on their prey and swimmers, but they rarely attack humans, so try not to panic. The great barracuda, the only barracuda species known to attack humans, can grow to 2 m (6 feet) long and weigh 45 kg (100 pounds).

Barracudas, like sharks, are attracted to surface splashing, underwater commotion, and reflective jewelry on swimmers. Bites are managed as you would a shark bite (see "Sharks," facing page). Embedded teeth may be found in the wound.

Moray Eels

Sharp-toothed moray eels can inflict deep puncture wounds. To prevent these bites (which are defensive reactions when the eel is cornered or provoked), divers and snorkelers should avoid placing a hand in an unexplored crevice or cave, or beneath coral and rocks.

Puncture wounds result from the creature's long, sharp fanglike teeth and powerful jaws. If a person pulls away reflexively and abruptly after being bitten, underlying structures (nerves, blood vessels, tendons, and ligaments) can be cut. If possible, let the eel open its mouth by itself (which it will usually do) to prevent a deep, slashing laceration. Doing this requires nerves of steel.

Carefully inspect the wound for teeth fragments, debride, and irrigate with povidone-iodine (Betadine) solution. The risk of infection for hand, wrist, ankle, and foot wounds is quite high. Splint a punctured joint and administer prophylactic antibiotics. As with other puncture wounds, never suture or tape it closed.

Leeches

While attached to the skin and feeding, leeches inject a chemical to prevent blood clotting and promote bleeding. The leech falls off after feeding. The wounds develop large blisters and dead tissue, which heal slowly.

Do not attempt to tear a leech forcibly from the skin; first, apply vinegar, rubbing alcohol, or a hot match head near the site of attachment. Clean the wound several times daily with dilute povidone-iodine (Betadine) solution and check the wound for retained mouthparts.

Water Moccasins and Sea Snakes

Water moccasins (also known as cottonmouths), aquatic and land snakes native to the southeastern United States but now found around waters from Virginia to Florida, extending westward to central Texas, belong to the pit viper family. They have a characteristically triangular head, a deep pit (heat receptor organ) between the eye and nostril, and a catlike, elliptical pupil.

Sea snakes inhabit the western Pacific Ocean and the Indian Ocean, the waters around Hawaii, and the west coast of Central America and South America from Baja California to Ecuador. They are not found in the Atlantic Ocean or the Caribbean.

Water moccasins bite with two fangs, and sea snakes with four to twenty. The precise bite pattern varies and can be misleading in identifying the snake.

Signs and Symptoms

Signs and symptoms of a water moccasin's envenomation include burning pain immediately after the bite followed by swelling of the extremity over a period of 6 to 12 hours. The faster the swelling progresses, the worse the degree of envenomation. Blistering and bruising develop at the site, followed by numbness, tingling, and twitching of the lips and face within the first hour. Bleeding from the nose and mouth may develop after 6 to 12 hours.

The venom from a sea snake causes muscle and nerve damage and injures the blood cells. In contrast to the water moccasin bite, the wound is not painful. Serious envenomation produces symptoms within 2 to 3 hours. These include painful muscle movements, drooping eyelids, blurred vision, lockjaw, difficulty with swallowing and breathing, drowsiness, and paralysis. If symptoms do not develop within 6 to 8 hours, there has been no envenomation.

Treatment

Treat this emergency as you would a land snakebite (see "Venomous Snakebites," page 197). Never approach or touch a sea snake, dead or alive. Even a decapitated snake can reflexively bite and inject venom.

Crocodiles and Alligators

These fearsome reptiles are found in tropical areas throughout the world. The dangerous saltwater or estuarine crocodile is found in Australia, Papua New Guinea, Indonesia, Malaysia, the Solomon Islands, and Thailand. Their preferred habitat is in the tidal reaches of rivers (up to 161 km [100 miles] inland), saltwater estuaries, and coastal inlets with mangroves. They can grow to a length of 6 m (20 feet), swim up to 32 km/h (20 miles per hour), and charge short distances on land at a speed of 24 to 48 km/h (15 to 30 miles per hour). The Nile crocodile, found in Africa, is equally large and dangerous. American crocodiles and alligators are half the size, slower, and less prone to attack.

The best defense is to be on your guard. Don't swim, wade, or snorkel in crocodile territory. Stay a few meters (yards) back from the water's edge when walking, and avoid entering the water when beaching or launching your dinghy. Seek local advice about the threat of crocodiles in the area, and above all, never interfere with or approach a crocodile. Treatment for bites is the same as for shark bites (see "Sharks," page 264).

HAZARDOUS MARINE LIFE: CREATURES THAT CUT
Corals and Barnacles

These living animals inflict a seemingly minor injury that can easily become infected. As with all wounds acquired in the marine environment, these are often contaminated with seawater debris, slime, sand, bacteria, and other infectious agents.

To avoid infection from coral and barnacle cuts and scrapes, scrub the area vigorously with soap and fresh water, then flush the wound with a large amount of water. Use clean, disinfected fresh water (if available) or bottled drinking water. Remove any visible debris. Continue by flushing with a half-strength solution of hydrogen peroxide and water (the bubbling action helps bring debris to the surface). Rinse the area again with clean water. Apply antibiotic ointment and cover with a nonadherent dressing. Clean the wound twice a day. If the wound shows any sign of infection (increased redness, pus, swollen lymph glands, or red streaks near the wound), begin antibiotics such as cephalexin (Keflex), ciprofloxacin (Cipro), or levofloxacin (Levaquin).

HAZARDOUS MARINE LIFE: CREATURES THAT IRRITATE THE SKIN
Sponges

Contact with sponges can lead to a poison ivy–type reaction with redness, itching, and swelling. Treat the irritation by soaking the affected area with vinegar for 10 to 30 minutes three times a day. If vinegar is not available, apply a soak of rubbing alcohol for 5 minutes. Dry the skin and repeatedly apply and remove sticky adhesive tape (duct tape works) to the area to remove any embedded sponge spicules. Repeat the vinegar soak for 5 minutes, or apply rubbing alcohol for 1 minute. Apply 1% hydrocortisone cream twice daily until the irritation is resolved. Monitor for signs of infection and treat appropriately.

Sea Cucumbers

Treat any skin irritation resulting from contact with a sea cucumber the same as for a jellyfish sting (see "Jellyfish," page 256). If the eyes are involved, flush with at least 1 L (1 quart) of water.

Seaweed and Dermatitis

When offending algae are trapped beneath swimsuits, an itchy, burning red rash known as seaweed dermatitis may appear within minutes to hours after swimming. Vigorously scrub the skin with soap and water, rinse with copious amounts of fresh water, and then rinse with 40 to 70% isopropyl alcohol. Apply 1% hydrocortisone cream twice daily. Severe burning, pain, and blisters are signs of an allergic reaction, requiring oral prednisone (Deltasone and others) and antihistamines.

Schistosomes and Swimmer's Itch

Swimmer's itch is caused by freshwater parasites called schistosomes, which burrow into the skin as it dries after swimming. The initial symptom is a prickling sensation, followed by itching within an hour after drying. The rash, resembling mosquito bites, is found on the exposed areas of the swimmer. These areas may form tiny blisters and pustules, which persist for up to 2 weeks. Mild cases can be treated by application of 40% isopropyl alcohol or calamine lotion, while more severe cases require oral prednisone (Deltasone and others), administered like the tapering dose schedule for jellyfish stings (see "Jellyfish: Treatment," page 258). Topical or systemic antibiotics may be required to treat infection. To reduce skin exposure, a full-length protective suit is required. If in a bathing suit only, dry off briskly with a towel immediately after leaving the water.

Jellyfish and Anemone Larvae and Seabather's Eruption

The stings from the larvae of jellyfish and anemones cause stinging or burning of the skin underneath covered areas (bathing suit, swim fins, bathing cap) while swimming or immediately upon leaving the water. Surfers may develop a rash on the chest and abdomen in the areas of contact with the surfboard. Itchy, raised red bumps develop within minutes or up to 12 hours after exposure. The stings resemble insect bites and may progress to blisters and hives. Decontamination and treatment are similar to those for jellyfish stings (see "Jellyfish," page 256). Try meat tenderizer (papain) if available; it may be more effective than vinegar. Swimwear should be washed with detergent and heat-dried before wearing again to prevent recurrent stinging of adherent larvae.

Erysipelothrix (Fish-Handler's Disease)

When small nicks and cuts on the hands of people cleaning fish and shellfish become infected with the bacterium *Erysipelothrix*, a distinctive skin rash develops. It appears up to a week after exposure as a sharply defined red-to-violet circular area of raised skin surrounding the wound. It is slightly warm and tender, and generally spreads on the top of the hand and between adjacent fingers. Treatment with antibiotics is necessary. Amoxicillin clavulanate (Augmentin) or ciprofloxacin (Cipro) should be administered for 7 to 10 days (see also "Erysipelothrix [Fish-Handler's Disease]," page 149).

SEAFOOD POISONING

Scombroid Poisoning

Scombroid poisoning results from eating fish that have undergone bacterial decomposition because of improper refrigeration. This breakdown process commonly occurs with fish having dark (brown or red) flesh, such as albacore, anchovies, sardines, herring, bluefin and yellowfin tuna, wahoo, bonito, mahimahi (dorado, or school dolphin), mackerel, dolphin (Hawaii), and bluefish (coastal New England). The illness can also arise from eating canned, smoked, and frozen fish improperly refrigerated prior to processing. Affected fish may smell of ammonia and often have a metallic, sharp, or peppery taste; some, however, may be normal in color and flavor. Cooking will not destroy the toxins.

Within 15 to 90 minutes after eating the fish, symptoms similar to an allergic reaction develop rapidly. These symptoms may include flushing of the face, neck, and chest (made worse with sun exposure); itching; hives; abdominal pain; nausea; vomiting; diarrhea; a low-grade fever; headache; and a variety of other symptoms, including shortness of breath, wheezing, palpitations, and feeling light-headed because of falling blood pressure. Left untreated, symptoms often resolve in 8 to 12 hours. Treat mild reactions with diphenhydramine (Benadryl) 25 to 50 mg every 4 to 6 hours; an alternative treatment is ranitidine (Zantac) or cimetidine (Tagamet) every 12 hours alone or with diphenhydramine. If a large amount of fish has been consumed within the previous hour, and the person is not having difficulty breathing, administer 50 g of activated charcoal (Actidose). (Charcoal binds toxins and prevents more from being absorbed.) Severe reactions

require treatment as described for anaphylactic shock (see "Anaphylactic Shock," page 37).

Prevention
- Scombroid poisoning can be prevented by storing fish at 15°C
  (59°F) or lower.
- Gut and place on ice any fish caught for consumption.
- Do not eat fish left in the sun for more than 2 hours.
- Carefully check the freshness of any fish purchased, especially if
  you suspect it was not packed in ice after being caught. If the fish
  has a dull appearance, lacks a sheen or oily rainbow appearance,
  or carries the odor of ammonia, do not consume it.

Ciguatera Poisoning

Ciguatera is the most common nonbacterial seafood-related illness. It
is found in the bottom-feeding reef fishes in the South Pacific, Indian
Ocean, Caribbean, and especially the coastal waters of Hawaii and
Florida. Ciguatoxin concentrates up the food chain as small reef fish
consume toxin-producing tiny organisms (dinoflagellates of the species *Gambierdiscus toxicus*), and larger reef fish eat the contaminated
smaller fish. Think of the "B-A-G-S" fish carrying the greatest risk for
ciguatera: barracuda, amberjack, grouper, and snapper. Other contaminated predatory fish include mullet and kingfish. In Hawaii, parrot fish
and surgeonfish predominate. The toxin does not impart any unusual
appearance or odor to the fish, nor is it inactivated by cooking, marinat-
ing, smoking, or freezing. The taste may be normal or metallic.

The first symptoms are usually experienced within 3 hours following ingestion, sometimes within 15 to 30 minutes. Symptoms include
diarrhea, nausea, vomiting, and abdominal pain. Other symptoms are
headache; itching; chills; numbness and tingling around the mouth,
tongue, and throat; a metallic taste; fatigue; debilitating weakness;
muscle and joint aches; and a variety of odd symptoms that may
appear after a delay of several days and last for months. The most
distinctive symptom is the reversal of hot and cold temperature perception; a cold beverage may feel like it is burning the lips and tongue,
and a warm breeze may be chilling. Death occurs from abnormal heart
rhythms and respiratory paralysis in up to 12 percent of those affected.

If the person is alert and breathing normally, administer 50 g of activated charcoal (Actidose).

Mild cases can be treated with diphenhydramine (Benadryl) or other antihistamines to relieve itching, and acetaminophen (Tylenol) for headache. There is no standard treatment or cure, therefore prevention is critical.

Immunity does not occur after exposure to the toxin. Relapses occur when again eating even a small amount of contaminated fish, and the reaction may be more severe. Ingestion of alcohol may precipitate a recurrence of the symptoms even months after the illness.

Prevention
- Identify the fish you catch.
- It is generally safe to eat pelagic (open ocean) fish caught offshore, such as tuna, dolphin, and wahoo, which do not carry the toxin.
- Consume coastal small reef fish no larger than a dinner plate, or larger than 2 kg (5 pounds).
- Avoid all barracuda.
- Avoid eating fish after a large reef disturbance (storm, tsunami).
- Avoid the head, roe, and guts (where the toxin is concentrated) of all fish.
- Avoid eating fish caught in areas known to be contaminated; ask for and heed the advice of local fishers.

Puffer Fish Poisoning
Puffer fish and related species have a distinctive appearance—using air or seawater, they can inflate their bodies to a nearly spherical shape. A deadly toxin is concentrated in the skin and organs of the fish. Raw filets with minute amounts of toxin are served as a delicacy (fugu) in some countries; the diner experiences pleasant tingling sensations of the lips and tongue. Poisoning begins with the rapid onset of abdominal pain, vomiting, and diarrhea, followed by muscle weakness and paralysis. Death from shock and respiratory failure occurs in 60 percent of the people who eat puffer fish, usually within the first 6 hours of illness.

Treatment consists of advanced life-support measures. Minor poisoning should be closely monitored for later respiratory problems.

Advice Regarding Edible Fish

- Learn to identify species of fish.
- Eat only the flesh of fish, not the organs or head.
- If it doesn't look like a fish, don't eat it.
- Don't eat fish with parrot-shaped beaks.
- Don't eat fish with a boxlike shape.
- Don't eat fish with spines or bristles.
- Don't eat fish with silvery, torpedo-shaped bodies and a large, V-shaped tail.
- Don't eat fish with a head larger than the body.
- Don't eat fish with the ability to inflate the body with air or seawater.
- Don't eat fish with bad odor, indented flesh or skin, or sunken eyes.
- If the fish tastes bad, or burns or stings the tongue, discard it.
- Seek the advice of local fishers, but remember, they're not infallible.

Paralytic Shellfish Poisoning (PSP) and Other Shellfish-Related Illnesses

A variety of toxin-producing algae grow rapidly in the warmer waters of summer. Their mass can become so large that they discolor the water, producing pink, red, yellow, and other colored "tides." Some algae blooms may be colorless. These biological toxins concentrate in clams, oysters, scallops, mussels, and other shellfish, through their normal process of filtering large quantities of seawater. These contaminated shellfish cause severe illness when eaten either cooked or raw.

Symptoms of PSP begin with tingling and numbness inside and around the mouth within minutes of ingestion. These sensations spread rapidly to the neck, hands, and feet. Over 12 hours, weakness, drooling, difficulty speaking and swallowing, and progressive muscle paralysis develop; the person is unable to move or breathe. Administer activated charcoal (Actidose) if the person is awake and able to swallow. Rescue breathing may be necessary for the paralyzed person (who is also conscious!) while awaiting medical assistance.

Prevention includes knowledge of the shellfish areas and seasons that are safe for harvesting. Heed any posted warnings of closed shellfish areas. Avoid eating shellfish in coastal waters where there are numerous dead fish, seabirds, or marine mammals near shore; this may be an indicator of PSP toxins in the waters nearby.

A different toxin causes diarrheic shellfish poisoning. This illness causes abdominal cramps, nausea, vomiting, and diarrhea within 2 hours after ingestion of the toxin. The symptoms will slowly resolve. Treatment consists of rehydrating the person.

Other identified toxins in shellfish may become airborne in the coastal winds, producing tearing of the eyes, a runny nose, and wheezing, similar to an allergic reaction.

Bacteria and viruses in the marine environment are also concentrated in shellfish. Contaminated shellfish, especially when eaten raw or undercooked, can cause a variety of gastrointestinal illnesses with diarrhea, fever, abdominal cramps, nausea, vomiting, and severe dehydration. When cooking shellfish, continue cooking for at least 5 minutes after the shell opens.

Obtain medical consultation for any severe illness persisting for more than 36 hours, or if the condition worsens (see "When to Worry: Diarrhea," page 174). Treat according to the guidelines for treatment of diarrhea.

HOW TO ABANDON SHIP

Before abandoning ship, the first priority is to dress warmly and put on a life jacket. Put on a survival suit or layer on as much warm, quick-drying clothing as possible. Broadcast a Mayday on available radios using VHF-FM channel 16 (effective up to a 32-km [20-mile] range) and SSB 2182 kHz. Repeat the ship's location slowly and distinctly, and monitor VHF channel 16 on a handheld radio for a response. If you have a satellite phone, make calls to designated rescue coordination centers in the area (you should have these numbers in the emergency ditch bag and in the boat's radio station). Activate a 406-MHz emergency position-indicating radio beacon (EPIRB), leave it on, and designate someone to bring it into the raft. A 406-MHz EPIRB must be registered with NOAA. (This can be done online at www.beaconregistration.noaa.gov.) Failure to register your beacon will likely delay the launch of a rescue mission.

Utilize appropriate visual distress signals if another vessel is in sight. Simultaneously, other crew should launch the life raft and locate the abandon ship bag (a survival kit). It is recommended to augment the modest amount of survival gear found in most life rafts by having select items packed inside the raft container at the time of its annual repack (include VHF radio, EPIRB, water maker, medical kit, signal pack, and sharp knives). These items can also be packed into a waterproof bag and secured by a short line to the raft canister.

Each crew member should have an easily accessible waterproof bag containing extra dry clothing, personal medications, passport, prescription eyeglasses and sunglasses, personal strobe, safety harness and tether, wallet, and any other personal valuables (including this book). Take jerry jugs of fresh water (two-thirds full so they float), extra food (especially carbohydrates), and navigation tools.

Attach the line coming out of the canister (painter) to the boat before the raft is inflated to prevent it from drifting away. To launch the raft, throw the canister or bag overboard on the downwind (leeward) side of the boat and then give a sharp jerk on the outstretched painter. This triggers the CO_2 cartridge and inflates the raft. If the first pull is unsuccessful, give it a stronger tug.

Once everyone is aboard, get away from the sinking vessel by quickly paying out all the painter line. Be prepared to cut the painter should the ship begin to sink after the crew has entered the raft.

If the vessel remains afloat, attach a quick-release line to it. The wreckage is always easier to spot than a small life raft and remains a source of additional food and supplies.

When possible, try to remain dry and enter the raft directly from the sinking boat rather than from the water. If you must enter cold water, ease yourself in to avoid the cold shock response. Use the automatically deployed boarding ladder and handholds at the entrance to the raft. Get everyone out of the water quickly. If you swim away from the raft to help a crewmate, be certain that you are attached to the raft with a safety line.

The hissing sound heard after inflation does not signify a leaking or defective raft. The relief valve is simply releasing excess gas pressure. Beginning immediately after the release of the CO_2/nitrogen mixture into the raft's interior space, ventilate the life raft thoroughly and periodically thereafter. Inflate the floor separately with the manual pump to provide insulation from the cold sea. Because the craft is vulnerable to capsize, it is important to inventory and secure all equipment as it comes aboard. Check the life raft for damage and leaks, and check the crew for serious injuries.

The first medical action is distribution of seasickness medication. Everyone in a life raft is susceptible to seasickness, especially in the first 24 hours. Bail the raft and remove wet clothing. Close the door, and huddle together to conserve heat. Do everything possible to conserve body heat, strength, and spirit, and prepare for rescue.

Life rafts have ballast pockets under the floor to trap seawater and increase stability. Capsize is most likely immediately after launching, when the raft is empty. If practical, have one or two of the fittest, heaviest crew board the raft early to provide additional stability and to ensure that the ballast water pockets are filling. They can also assist in transferring equipment and helping others into the raft.

No immediate danger exists if the raft capsizes with crew inside, since sufficient air is available in the space under the canopy. It is necessary to enter the water in order to right the raft, since it is unlikely to right itself unless rolled again by successive waves. With the raft empty, it can be righted by pulling on the righting straps at the bottom. Kneel on the downwind side with feet braced on the CO_2 cylinder, and lean back. The raft will right itself easily when the wind catches it.

To prevent recurrent capsizes in heavy winds and seas, use the cone-shaped sea anchor. Stream the sea anchor after the raft is clear of the sinking vessel, and protect the raft from chafe at the point where the rope is attached. Weight distribution is critical to avoid capsize. Position most of the crew on the windward side (side facing the wind, and the same side from which the sea anchor is deployed) to act as ballast. This reduces the chance of the raft being overturned by the wind. In rough seas, be prepared to maintain the raft's balance, and quickly shift weight as needed to prevent capsize. Whenever a raft capsizes, gather the crew in the water and check that no one is under the raft. Reenter quickly to avoid the progression of the cold shock response and to conserve precious energy.

Preparation for Rescue: Life in the Raft

After abandoning ship and securing crew and equipment in the raft, prepare for rescue. Panic, fear, helplessness, and hopelessness can defeat the best-equipped and most experienced crew. Crews that are optimistic are likely to survive. Leaders set the example and improve morale by staying calm and formulating an active strategy to be rescued. Assigning meaningful duties to everyone by structuring work and rest time instills in the crew some sense of control over their destiny.

Most people who abandon ship near populated coastal areas or shipping lanes around the world, or perhaps anywhere on the planet, are likely to be rescued, or at least have a rescue vessel or aircraft deployed, within 24 to 72 hours if they have activated an EPIRB registered with NOAA and are able to use additional radios and satellite phones. Communication has now become the keystone to survival."

The Alaska Marine Safety Education Association (AMSEA) has compiled the following "Seven Steps to Survival":

1. Recognition: Recognize you are in a survival situation.
2. Inventory: Inventory your equipment.
3. Shelter: Create and maintain a shelter.
4. Signals
5. Water
6. Food
7. Attitude

After entering the raft, review how to use the distress signals. Inventory the signaling devices available, and agree on priorities for use. Be sure the EPIRB is turned on, and leave it on. Battery life is 48 hours.

Maintain continuous lookout for rescue boats and airplanes, and rotate the watch schedule every 2 hours. Other duties include medical care and comfort to injured and ill persons, making drinking water, organizing the stores, keeping the log, bailing, and maintaining the raft.

Protect the raft against sharp, pointed, and abrasive objects, such as knives, tools, fishhooks, spears, fish bones and teeth, shells, belt buckles, jewelry, and pens. Keep all pointed tools sheathed or wrapped except when in use.

After seasickness, no other condition is more debilitating than chronic sleep deprivation. Whenever possible, lie down and rest. Insulate the recumbent body against heat loss, especially from the cold floor of the raft. Keep the double bottom of the floor fully inflated, and make every effort to keep the raft dry (hypothermia, rather than exposure to severe weather, is perhaps the greatest threat to survival). Line the floor with sails, tarps, and extra clothing. The double-layer floor also protects against the bumps of sharks, dorado, and other fish.

Spraying saltwater directly on the skin or clothing to cool the body in tropical climates is not helpful. Salt-encrusted skin is likely to break down and become infected. Dry clothing protects the skin from painful saltwater boils and other bacterial infections. Apply an emollient to knees, hands, elbows, and buttocks to decrease skin abrasion. Put antibiotic cream on areas of skin breakdown, and cover with a dry dressing.

Recognition of the early signs of hypothermia is critical. Prompt treatment usually prevents progression to severe hypothermia, which is fatal, since it is untreatable in the raft. Treatment of mild to moderate hypothermia consists of preventing further heat loss by sheltering the person from the wind, sea spray, and rain. Remove wet clothing and dry the skin completely, then dress the person in multiple layers of dry clothing. If a change of clothing is impossible, provide a vapor barrier with foul-weather gear. If a blanket is available, wrap the person like a burrito, covering the head, neck, and face. Let the person shiver; if shivering is vigorous, the heat generated internally provides the most effective method of rewarming. Calories from carbohydrates, and ample water, provide the fuel necessary for the muscles to continue shivering.

Foil space blankets made of aluminized Mylar are useful as sun reflectors on the canopy, and they effectively minimize heat loss through radiation. When wrapped in the blanket, body heat loss is reduced by 80 to 90 percent.

To prevent heat-related illness and dehydration, drink water at regular intervals. If possible, keep drinking until the urine is clear. (Mechanisms for obtaining water are discussed later in this section.)

In tropical climates, keep clothing on to help reduce fluid loss. Clothing protects skin from sunburn and reduces passive heating from solar radiation. Apply sunscreen to exposed areas of the face, hands, arms, neck, and feet. Stay in the shade of the raft canopy, but make sure the raft is well-ventilated. Space blankets with a reflective surface may also be tied over the canopy to reflect the sun's rays. Deflating the raft's floor chambers helps to cool the raft. It may be tempting to take a dip in cool seawater if you feel very hot. Be sure there is no hazardous marine life in the area and that you have the strength and ability to climb back aboard; post an alert lookout.

Depending on the outside temperature, the average person can survive approximately 10–12 days without a supply of fresh water; however, they will remain fit for only 5 to 6 days and will then become delirious. Dehydration causes significant deterioration in mental and physical performance. By contrast, complete starvation leads to death in 40 to 60 days if there is enough fresh drinking water. Reducing activity to a minimum will decrease the requirement for food and water. The evaporative loss from the action of sunlight in an open boat in the tropics is estimated at 2.5 L (5 pints) per day if the body is at rest.

Life rafts, if they contain any water rations, generally carry 1 L (1 quart) per person in 125-mL (½-cup) caches; some rafts include as little as a pint per person. It is recommended that "castaways" should restrict daily water intake to about 0.5 L (1 pint), unless supplies are plentiful. However, this is not the absolute minimal requirement. The critical amount of water for survival is 110 to 220 mL (½ cup to 1 cup) per day. This is not the amount to support health and vigor! Consumption of less than 110 mL (½ cup) per day increases the risk of death.

Hand-operated, portable, reverse-osmosis desalination units produce 220 ml (1 cup) of water in 15 minutes and can hydrate as many as 25 individuals indefinitely if operated continuously. Rainwater can be collected with the canopy of the life raft. An exterior gutter collects and routes the water to a large container for storage. Daily washing of the canopy with seawater whenever practical helps to remove the buildup of salt deposits.

Life-raft rations are similar to energy bars. Regard these as more of a medicine than a meal. Do not eat dry food unless water is available. With 2 L (2 quarts) of fresh water available daily, eat as desired. Fish and other sea creatures contain water with extremely low salt content in their eyes, flesh, and cerebrospinal fluid. Fish blood has a high salt concentration and is not recommended. Juices can be pressed out of the flesh by twisting pieces of fish in a cloth. The blood from seabirds and turtles is also a reliable source of hydration for castaways.

Seawater is not drinkable, yet intolerable thirst may drive castaways to drink it. Succumbing to this temptation is a major cause of death. Drinking seawater usually causes immediate vomiting.

In high latitudes, old sea ice is a good source of water. Sea ice loses its salt content after a year. The ice is brittle, bluish in color, and has round edges. New sea ice is gray, salty, opaque, and hard. Melting ice allows for tasting and judging the salinity. If the temperature drops to freezing, seawater can be collected in a can and allowed to freeze. Fresh water freezes first. Therefore, the salt concentrates in the center, forming slush surrounded by ice containing very little salt. Sea ice should not be confused with ice in an iceberg. Water from melted iceberg chunks is fresh, drinkable water.

Unless survivors are assured of an early rescue or have a water maker, they should consume no water in the first 24 hours and utilize the body's reserves. Thereafter, restrict intake to about 0.5 L (1 pint) a day. If water is plentiful, drink up to a 1 L (1 quart) or so daily. Plan to eat very little for the first 3 days. Thereafter, begin the lifeboat rations of carbohydrates. Save some until rescue is imminent, when you will need extra energy.

Fish are usually the mainstay of a diet at sea. The raft casts a dark shadow beneath the surface, which appears as a safe haven for a variety of fish, especially dorado. Fish can be taken near the sea surface with a harpoon, gaff, or speargun. The ideal area to strike is located just behind the gill cover. Attach all fishing gear to the raft with a lanyard to avoid losing it. Trailing a line with a baited hook can catch fish far from the raft. Bait can be obtained by using the guts, stomach contents, or thin strips of flesh from the first fish caught. Lures can be made from any shiny object.

At night, fish are attracted to bright lights. Instead of a flashlight, try a signal mirror or any other shiny surface to reflect moonlight onto the water.

When bringing a fish aboard the raft, use a cloth to wrap the fish. Dolphin and wahoo both have serrated teeth and thrash wildly out of the water. Have a cutting surface ready to kill fish quickly by cutting through the spine behind the head. Large fish can be stunned with a blow to the top of the head at eye level, and simply covering its eyes will calm it down sufficiently to position it for a quick kill.

To save fish for future meals, cut the flesh into thin strips about 2.5 cm (1 inch) wide and 1 cm (0.5 inch) thick, and spread them out to dry in the sun on a flat surface. Fish spoils within hours in the heat, so start drying some as soon as it is caught. Most ocean fish can safely be eaten raw.

All kelp and almost all brown and green (not red) seaweed are edible. If it tastes bitter, it may be one of the rare poisonous varieties.

Every effort should be made to avoid attracting sharks. Take special care to dispose of blood and offal at night, preferably when the raft is moving. Try not to create a waste trail for the sharks to follow, and bring hooked or speared fish aboard as quickly as possible.

All seabirds are edible, but catching them involves more luck than skill. Float a baited hook on the water (fish guts are best), and let the bird hook itself. After the bird is hooked, throw a piece of canvas or article of clothing over the bird and compress the chest to suffocate it. The forewings and legs make excellent bait, and the feathers can be made into fishing lures.

PREPARING FOR FOREIGN TRAVEL AND EXTENDED WORLD CRUISING

Nearly one-half of travelers to developing countries become ill during their visit. Diseases, such as polio, malaria, and typhoid fever, that are uncommon in the United States are a threat to travelers who visit areas where poor sanitation and contaminated food and water exist. International travelers should contact their local health department, physician, or travel medicine clinic at least 6 weeks prior to departure, to obtain current health information on countries they plan to visit and to begin receiving vaccinations. Beside vaccinations, travelers should undergo medical and dental physical exams prior to departure and obtain prescription medications that might be needed during travel (see Appendix B, page 297).

Motor vehicle accidents are a major health problem for travelers. (They are the most common cause of death for Peace Corps workers.) A large contributory factor is the confusion and lack of experience for those who come from left-side driving countries to right-side driving countries, and vice versa, as are the distractions attendant to driving in new and unfamiliar areas. In addition, seat belts may not be available, and taxi and bus drivers may not be skilled and experienced. If the vehicle's condition is poor, don't risk riding in it. Whenever possible, avoid vehicular travel at night. Alcohol is often a contributory factor.

Driving a rental motor scooter, and riding a bicycle on narrow highways and local streets, can be especially hazardous. Consider purchasing a supplemental "medical assistance" insurance policy.

The Centers for Disease Control and Prevention (CDC) Travelers' Health website (www.cdc.gov/travel) provides help in locating clinics for pretravel consultation. The Travel Clinics page also provides links to state health departments and facilities approved to provide yellow fever vaccinations.

The CDC website also provides travel health information to address the many different health risks a traveler may face, along with information to assist travelers in deciding the vaccines, medications, and other measures necessary to prevent illness and injury during international travel. *CDC Health Information for International Travel* (The Yellow Book) is the most trusted resource for travel health and is available in a searchable online version at www.cdc.gov/yellowbook.

The World Health Organization (WHO) also maintains recommendations regarding vaccine requirements for international travelers, with its annual publication of vaccination requirements and health advice at www.who.int/ith.

Timing of Vaccines

Acquisition of vaccinations should begin at least 6 weeks prior to departure. Travelers often request vaccinations at the last minute, leading to concerns about the appropriate timing and spacing of injections. In general, inactivated vaccines or toxoids, such as those for hepatitis B, cholera, typhoid, rabies, plague, influenza, tetanus, diphtheria, or inactivated polio, may be given simultaneously at separate sites.

Live vaccines, such as those for measles, mumps, rubella, and oral polio, can be administered simultaneously with an inactivated vaccine, except those for cholera and yellow fever. Immune globulin given for hepatitis A can be given simultaneously with inactivated vaccines and toxoids. Live vaccines should be given at least 2 weeks before immune globulin or 3 to 5 months afterward.

Required Vaccines

Yellow fever (YF) is an acute viral hemorrhagic disease transmitted to humans by mosquitoes in tropical Africa and South America. YF transmission occurs in jungle and urban areas in South America, with peak transmission during the months of January through March.

Countries located in YF-endemic areas, such as some African countries (Burkina Faso, Cameroon, Congo, Côte D'Ivoire, Democratic Republic of Congo, Gabon, Ghana, Liberia, Mali, Mauritania, Niger, Rwanda, São Tomé, Togo) and one in South America (French Guiana), require proof of YF vaccination from all arriving travelers.

The vaccine is a live attenuated virus. The immunization must be given no less than 10 days prior to planned date of entry. Vaccine administration is documented and stamped on the appropriate page of the International Certificate of Vaccination. This proof of vaccination is sometimes required during crossing of international borders, particularly in Africa, or if flying from an infected country to a noninfected country, even if the stay in the endemic country was a brief transit stop.

YF vaccine is approved for use in all persons over 9 months of age who have no YF vaccine contraindication. The primary schedule for YF vaccine in adults is a single 0.5-mL injection given subcutaneously. The duration of immunity from one dose of the vaccine is estimated to last for 10 years or longer. A booster dose is recommended for persons with continued risk of exposure 10 years from the last dose.

YF vaccine can be administered concurrently or at any time before or after immune globulin products given for hepatitis A prophylaxis.

Recommended Vaccines

Diphtheria, measles, mumps, rubella, and polio are childhood immunizations that all international travelers should keep up-to-date. Tetanus should be updated with a booster every 10 years. Travelers born after 1956, who have not received two doses of measles vaccine or do not have a well-documented history of having the illness as a child, should receive a single injection of the measles vaccine. Travelers who have previously completed a primary polio series and have never had a booster should receive a booster dose of oral polio vaccine (OPV). Further information on this can be found on the World Health Organization website (www.who.int/vaccines/GlobalSummary/Immunization/CountryProfileSelect.cfm). Cases of measles and chickenpox have been reported as travel-acquired infections among international travelers, and these common childhood infectious diseases are known to cause more serious disease in infections acquired by adults.

Cholera Vaccine

The highest incidence of cholera cases in the world is being reported in Africa, predominantly South Africa, Democratic Republic of the Congo, Mozambique, and Malawi.

Cholera vaccine is not required for entry into any country under current WHO International Health Regulations, and it is not recommended for short-term tourists traveling to an endemic country. Immunization may be recommended for travelers who plan extensive travel or work in highly endemic/epidemic areas under unsanitary conditions and without access to Western-style medical care.

The newer cholera vaccines are the live attenuated oral vaccines and killed whole cell (KWC) oral vaccines. The live attenuated oral cholera CVD 103-HgR vaccine is extremely safe. The vaccine should not be given to immunosuppressed people or those with chronic liver disease. There are no data on safety in pregnant women. The killed whole cell oral cholera vaccine also appears to be extremely safe; the only contraindication is intolerance to a previously administered dose.

The KWC vaccine is taken in 2 doses separated by 7 to 42 days. A booster is recommended every 2 years for repeated exposure.

Hepatitis A Vaccine

Hepatitis A is a viral infection transmitted by contaminated food or water or even by direct person-to-person contact. Hepatitis A is one of the most common vaccine-preventable infections acquired during travel. The risk of hepatitis A infection is highest in developing countries with poor sanitation and food hygiene. Most travel-related cases (72 percent) are associated with travel to Mexico, Central America, and South America.

Hepatitis A vaccine (Havrix) is recommended for travelers going to developing countries where sanitation may be poor. The vaccine is given as a single injection to adults and as 2 injections 1 month apart to children under 17 years of age. A booster injection 6 to 12 months later is also recommended. It takes at least 3 weeks to be protected after the initial injection. Travelers who arrive in a high-risk area less than 3 weeks from the date of their vaccination should also receive hepatitis immune globulin. A single injection of immune globulin is protective for up to 5 months, depending on the dose. Immune globulin prepared in the United States carries no risk of transmission of AIDS. It is also safe to use during pregnancy.

Hepatitis B Vaccine

Although hepatitis B (HB) vaccine was incorporated into the schedule of routine childhood immunizations starting in the late 1980s, HB vaccine is a recommended travel vaccine for certain susceptible adult travelers who are going to areas where the disease is endemic.

Indications

The HB vaccine is recommended for travelers who anticipate exposure to blood or body secretions (health care personnel, relief workers), unprotected sexual exposures with members of the local population or others, and adventure travelers who are at higher risk of accidents and needing medical attention.

Dosing Schedule

For adults, the dose of the HB vaccine is 1.0 mL given intramuscularly in the deltoid muscle. The primary immunization schedule consists of 3 vaccine doses given on a schedule of 0, 1, and 6 months. The vaccine should be given intramuscularly for best response, but HB vaccine should not be given in the buttock, because this route of administration has been associated with a lower immune response.

Accelerated Schedule

The 3-dose primary series may be accelerated to be administered at 0, 1, and 4 months, or 0, 2, and 4 months, where the second dose should be given at least 1 month after the first dose, and the third dose should be given at least 4 months after the first dose, and at least 2 months after the second dose.

Japanese Encephalitis Vaccine

Japanese encephalitis (JE) is a mosquito-transmitted virus infection that is endemic in Asia and potentially fatal. In temperate regions the transmission season generally extends from April through November, with a peak in July through September. In tropical or subtropical regions of Oceania and Southeast Asia, transmission may occur year-round.

Indications

Decisions regarding the use of JE vaccine for travel must balance the low risk for disease and the small chance of an adverse event following immunization. JE vaccine should be considered by travelers who plan to spend a month or longer in endemic areas, particularly in rural areas, during the transmission season. Travelers planning extensive unprotected outdoor, evening, and nighttime exposure in rural areas may be at risk even if the trip is very short. Risk of transmission is higher in rural areas, especially where pigs are raised and where rice fields, marshes, and standing pools of water provide breeding grounds for mosquitoes and feed for birds.

Dosing Schedule

For travelers older than 3 years, the recommended primary schedule in adults is a series of 3 doses of 1.0 mL of JE-VAX administered by subcutaneous injection on a schedule of 0, 7, and 30 days. The immunity should last for at least 3 years after primary immunization series.

Meningococcal Vaccine

Neisseria meningitidis spreads through the air via droplets of contaminated respiratory secretions or through person-to-person contact (kissing, sharing cigarettes and drinking glasses, etc.).

Indications

Meningococcal vaccine is recommended for travelers to some countries of Africa during the dry season from December through June, especially if prolonged contact with the local populace is likely. Those countries include Benin, Burkina Faso, Cameroon, Central African

Republic, Chad, Côte D'Ivoire, Djibouti, Ethiopia, Gambia, Ghana, Guinea, Guinea-Bissau, Mali, Niger, Nigeria, Senegal, Sudan, Somalia, and Togo.

Dosing Schedule
The quadrivalent meningococcal polysaccharide vaccine consists of a single dose of 0.5 mL by subcutaneous injection to adults. This vaccine should be administered 1 to 2 weeks before departure.

Adverse Events
Minor side effects, consisting of local pain, swelling, redness of the skin at the site of injection, and, rarely, a low-grade fever, have been reported.

Rabies Vaccine
Preexposure vaccination against rabies is recommended for travelers to endemic areas who are at increased risk, such as veterinarians, animal handlers, spelunkers, and biologists. A series of 3 injections over 3 weeks is required.

Typhoid Vaccine
Typhoid fever is an infection transmitted by contaminated food and water. High-risk areas for contracting this illness include southern Asia; the Middle East; East, West, and Central Africa; and Central and South America.

Although an injectable vaccine is still available, the newer oral typhoid vaccine is preferable. Both vaccines protect 50 to 80 percent of recipients.

- *Typhoid injectable vaccine:* This consists of 2 injections given at least 4 weeks apart. It is good for 3 years. It is about 70 percent effective in preventing the disease and is usually associated with 1 or 2 days of postinjection side effects. These include discomfort at the site of injection, fever, headache, and flu-like symptoms.
- *Oral typhoid vaccine:* This consists of four doses of one capsule, each given 2 days apart. The last dose should be given at least 1 week before travel to allow the vaccine time to work. A booster is required every 7 years. Adverse reactions are uncommon.

DISEASES OF SPECIAL INTEREST TO CRUISING SAILORS AND GLOBAL TRAVELERS

Malaria

Malaria is an infection of the bloodstream caused by a parasite transmitted to humans through the bite of the *Anopheles* mosquito. After a period ranging from a week to months, a flu-like illness develops, characterized by recurrent fevers, chills, headache, weakness, and lethargy. Fever in a traveler who has returned from a malaria-endemic area should be attributed to malaria until proven otherwise. More than 300 million people are infected each year, with 2 million to 3 million deaths; thus, it is a significant health threat to travelers.

Prevention

The best way to prevent malaria is to avoid mosquitoes. The *Anopheles* mosquito feeds at night. Thus, maximum precautions should be taken from dusk to dawn. It takes only one bite from an infected mosquito to acquire the disease. Wear thin, loose clothing that covers the arms and legs. At dusk, tuck your pants into your socks or shoes, and tape the cuffs of your shirtsleeves closed. Screens over portholes and the companionway, mosquito nets, and repellents should be used at night. When possible, anchor out and away from the shore, in a breezy area, and avoid walking the shore at dusk.

The most effective repellents contain 10 to 35 percent DEET (N, N-diethyl-toluamide). Children should use preparations with no more than 30 percent. There is little increase in protection from using stronger concentrations. The duration of action is between 2 and 6 hours, depending on the concentration of DEET, how much the wearer perspires, and how hungry the mosquito is. There have been rare case reports of adverse reactions to DEET, ranging from skin rashes to central nervous system (brain) disorders.

Picaridin is another effective chemical used in many mosquito repellents. Spraying or soaking clothing and bed nets with permethrin and letting them air-dry before use is also very helpful.

Antimalarial Drugs

All recommended preventive regimens involve taking a medicine before travel, during travel, and for a period of time after leaving the malaria-endemic area. Beginning the drug before travel allows the antimalarial agent to be in the blood before the traveler is exposed to malaria parasites and observe for any adverse reactions.

No antimalarial drug is absolutely effective. Travelers can still develop the disease regardless of how many medications they take. Tools such as the interactive CDC Malaria Map Application can assist in locating specific countries where malaria protection is needed (www.cdc.gov/malaria/map). Updated information can be obtained by referring to *CDC Health Information for International Travel* (The Yellow Book); the online version on the CDC Traveler's Health website at www.cdc.gov/yellowbook; or by phoning the CDC Malaria Hotline at 770-488-7788. Information on diagnosis and treatment of malaria is also available at www.cdc.gov/malaria.

The following drugs are used to prevent malaria:

- *Chloroquine:* There are only a few places left in the world where chloroquine is still effective in preventing malaria. Chloroquine is recommended for travel to Central America west of the Panama Canal Zone, Mexico, Haiti, the Dominican Republic, Egypt, and most countries in the Middle East (chloroquine resistance has been reported in Iran, Yemen, and Oman). The drug is generally safe, but side effects can include nausea, diarrhea, and upset stomach. It is taken once weekly, beginning 2 weeks prior to departure, continued weekly during travel in malaria areas, and for 4 weeks after leaving such areas.

- *Mefloquine:* Mefloquine is now the most widely prescribed drug for the prevention of malaria in parts of the world where the parasite is resistant to chloroquine. The adult dose is 250 mg once a week. The pediatric dose varies according to the weight of the child; check with your pediatrician. Mefloquine should be started 1 to 2 weeks before travel and continued for 4 weeks after leaving the endemic area. Mefloquine should not be taken during pregnancy, or while taking a beta-blocker or calcium channel blocker medication.

  Mefloquine can occasionally produce serious adverse reactions such as acute psychoses, hallucinations, anxiety, and seizures. Other side effects include nausea, upset stomach, and diarrhea.

- *Doxycycline (Vibramycin):* An alternative to mefloquine is doxycycline 100 mg daily, beginning 1 to 2 days before travel to malarious areas. This drug is not advised for pregnant women or children under 8 years of age. It can also cause a rash and severe sunburn in users exposed to the sun, and it is therefore a poor choice for sailors. Vaccination with the oral typhoid vaccine should be delayed for at least 24 hours after taking a dose of doxycycline.
- *Proguanil (Paludrine):* This drug may be used for malaria prevention where there is resistance to chloroquine. The adult dose is 200 mg daily along with weekly chloroquine.
- *Atovaquone and Proguanil (Malarone):* Atovaquone in combination with proguanil can be taken to prevent chloroquine-resistant malaria. The drug is taken at the same time each day with food or a milky drink. The drug should be started 2 days before entering a malaria-endemic area and continued for 7 days after return. The adult dose is 1 tablet (250 mg atovaquone/100 mg proguanil) per day. Malarone is very well-tolerated, and side effects are rare. The most common adverse effects are abdominal pain, nausea, and headache.
- *Pyrimethamine and Sulfadoxine (Fansidar):* Because of the drug's association with an unacceptably high incidence of toxic side effects when used for prevention, it is generally reserved only for treatment.

Latent Malaria

Certain forms of malaria *(Plasmodium vivax)* can hide in the liver and cause illness for as long as 4 years after returning from an endemic country. The drug primaquine, taken after the traveler has left a malaria area, can prevent this from occurring.

Treatment

Malaria can be treated effectively early in the course of the disease, but delay of therapy can have serious or fatal consequences. Travelers who have symptoms of malaria should seek medical evaluation as soon as possible. CDC recommendations for malaria treatment can be found at www.cdc.gov/malaria/diagnosis_treatment.

Consider self-treatment for a traveler who develops symptoms of malaria (fever, chills, and other flu-like symptoms) in a malaria-endemic country while not taking prophylactic malaria medicine, or who chose a suboptimal drug regimen (e.g., chloroquine in an area with chloroquine-resistant malaria). Consider atovaquone and proguanil (Malarone) for self-treatment if professional medical care is not available within 24 hours. Medical care should be sought immediately after treatment. The adult dose is 4 tablets (each dose contains 1000 mg atovaquone and 400 mg proguanil) orally as a single daily dose for 3 consecutive days.

Schistosomiasis

This is a parasitic disease transmitted by freshwater snails that excrete a parasite into the water. The parasite then penetrates the skin of humans during bathing or swimming in freshwater ponds, lakes, or rivers. The regions where schistosomiasis is most common include Brazil, Egypt, sub-Saharan Africa, southern China, the Philippines, and Southeast Asia.

Signs and Symptoms

Symptoms usually start 2 to 3 weeks after exposure and include fever, loss of appetite, abdominal pain, weakness, headaches, joint and muscle pain, diarrhea, nausea, cough, and itchy rash. Infection of the brain can produce seizures and visual loss.

Treatment

Praziquantel (Biltricide), an antiparasitic drug, will effectively cure the illness.

Dengue Fever

Dengue, primarily a disease of the tropics, is a very common mosquito-transmitted viral infection. It is now endemic in Asia, the South Pacific, the Caribbean basin, Mexico, Central America, South America, and Africa.

Prevention

The same mosquito that causes malaria also spreads this disease. Anyone who contracts a fever while traveling in malaria-infested areas should be tested for malaria before assuming the diagnosis is dengue fever. Travelers should follow mosquito avoidance measures (see "Malaria," page 288). No vaccine is available.

Signs and Symptoms

This viral illness ranges from a flu-like syndrome to a severe and fatal hemorrhagic disease. The milder infection begins with sudden fever, severe frontal headache, muscle and joint pain (so painful that the illness is sometimes called "breakbone fever"), fatigue, nausea and vomiting, and often a measles-like rash that appears 3 or 4 days after the fever. The rash appears as tiny red bumps that spread from the chest and back to the face, arms, and legs. The symptoms can be similar to and even mistaken for malaria.

The illness is usually self-limited and lasts about a week. Occasionally, a person will remain very weak for up to 1 month, or develop a severe and fatal syndrome called dengue hemorrhagic fever. There is no specific treatment, and a vaccine is not available.

The more severe and often fatal form of the disease progresses to generalized bleeding and shock. Most of these cases are reported in Southeast Asia, especially in children, and in people who have been repeatedly infected with the virus.

Treatment

Complete recovery takes 2 to 4 weeks. Control the fever with acetaminophen (Tylenol)—not aspirin, which may increase the risk of bleeding. If there is any evidence of bleeding, seek medical attention. There is no specific medication for dengue fever.

West Nile Virus

Mosquitoes transmit this virus, and birds are the most common reservoir.

Signs and Symptoms

The incubation period from bite to infection is 3 to 14 days. Most infections are asymptomatic or present with mild flu-like illness. Severe infections include meningitis and encephalitis.

Treatment
No specific treatment is available. Therapy is supportive.

Leptospirosis
Leptospirosis is caused by a spirochete that enters the body though the skin, eyes, mouth, or nose during swimming or bathing in fresh water. High-risk activities include rafting, kayaking, or swimming in fresh water.

Signs and Symptoms
After an incubation period of 7 to 12 days, infection causes high fever, headache, chills, muscle aches, and red eyes without exudate. After a few days, the infected person seems to recover, only to develop the return of less dramatic fever associated with relentless headache, and possibly jaundice and a red rash.

Treatment
The treatment of choice is doxycycline (Vibramycin) 100 mg twice a day for 7 days. Achromycin and others (tetracycline) 2 g in 4 divided doses for 7 to 14 days is an alternative.

There are three proven techniques for removing infectious organisms (bacteria, viruses, parasites) from water: filters, boiling, and chemical treatment.

Filters
Filters are commercially available with pore sizes small enough to remove *Giardia* organisms and most bacteria from water. Filters used to remove parasites should have an absolute (not nominal) pore size of 1 micron or smaller. This pore size is too large to remove viruses. After filtration, the water must be chemically treated to destroy viruses. Many filters now also contain iodine resins, which can kill viruses. New types of filters are effective for all classes of microorganisms. Using "Structured Matrix" technology, General Ecology (First Need Systems) has developed a filter that purifies water without chemical disinfectants. It is easily installed in the galley water system on a boat. Reverse-osmosis filters (water makers) are ideal for cruising sailors. They desalinate seawater and remove contaminating organisms, making the water pure and safe to drink, but only when stored in clean tanks.

Boiling
Much of the time required to bring water to a boil works toward disinfecting it. By the time it reaches boiling, the water is safe to drink. Although the boiling point of water decreases as altitude increases, this should not make a difference, since almost all organisms are killed well below the boiling point of water.

Chemicals
The two most common chemicals used to disinfect water are chlorine and iodine. Iodine is preferred over chlorine in the backcountry, because it

- is less affected by pH and nitrogenous wastes;
- imparts a taste that is better tolerated than that of chlorine;

■ is easier to transport;
■ can double as a topical disinfectant for wound care.

Iodine will not kill *Cryptosporidium* at concentrations used for disinfecting drinking water, and must be allowed to sit in the water for a longer period of time to kill *Giardia*.

Iodine takes longer to work in cold water, so the dose or the contact time with the water must be increased. Some iodine is absorbed by impurities in the water, so more is required for cloudy or polluted water. If you find the iodine taste objectionable, dissolving vitamin C (ascorbic acid) tablets or granules will help, but the treated water must not be used before enough time has elapsed for the microorganisms to be destroyed by the iodine. Artificial flavorings added to hide the taste often contain ascorbic acid, so observe the same precautions. To be safe, if you add flavoring of any kind, make sure to do so only after the iodine has had adequate contact time with the water.

Katadyn Micropur MP1 chlorine dioxide and Portable Aqua chlorine dioxide are easy-to-use, safe purification tablets. The chemical kills bacteria, viruses, *Cryptosporidium*, and *Giardia*, and it leaves no aftertaste. 1 tablet will treat 1 L (1 quart) of water.

Table 4: How to Use 10% Povidone-Iodine Solution (Betadine)

Water Temperature	Water Clarity	Drops per Liter or Quart	Contact Time
Warm	Clear	8	30 min.
Warm	Cloudy	16	30 min.
Cold (less than 10°C (50°F)	Clear	8	60 min.
Cold	Cloudy	16	60 min.
1 drop = .05 mL			

Table 5: How to Use Iodine Tablets

Water Temperature	Water Clarity	Tablets per Liter or Quart	Contact Time
Warm	Clear	1	15 min.
Warm	Cloudy	2	15 min.
Cold	Clear	1	45 min.
Cold	Cloudy	2	45 min.

Source: Data from H. Backer, "Field Water Disinfection," *Wilderness Medicine: Management of Wilderness and Environmental Emergencies*, 3rd edition. Edited by P.S. Auerbach (Mosby, 1995).

A quick way to purify water on a boat is to use ordinary household liquid bleach (Clorox), which contains 5.25% sodium hypochlorite and no other additives. Add 5 mL (1 teaspoon) of bleach for every 38 L (10 gallons) of water in the tank, and let stand for an hour. Using an activated charcoal filter in line with the galley faucet can eliminate the nasty taste of chlorine. The return of a chlorine taste will indicate that the filter is ready for replacement. Chlorine solutions are very unstable; chlorine is lost as the solution sloshes around while being transported. Replace stock solutions every 3 to 6 months. Treat smaller quantities of water as shown in **Table 6** (below).

Table 6: Sodium Hypochlorite (Bleach)

Drops per Liter or Quart	Water Temperature	Water Clarity	Contact Time
2	Warm	Clear	30 min
4	Warm	Cloudy	30 min
2	Cold	Clear	60 min
4	Cold	Cloudy	60 min
Note: Warm water is >15°C (60°F).			

Mix water well and let stand for 60 minutes. Keep an eyedropper taped to your emergency bottle of chlorine bleach.

Chlorine, like iodine, does not kill *Cryptosporidium* or amoebic cysts and is variably effective against *Giardia*. Install an appropriate water filtration system on the galley faucet for complete protection. If taking in water of suspect quality, double the amount of chlorine; also double the contact time if cold.

The vinyl hoses that are used in boat freshwater systems can become a serious source of contamination, even though the tanks have been cleaned. If the hose looks bad or discolored, replace it.

MARINE MEDICAL KITS

Thoughtful selection of the medical supplies presented here involves consideration of the following factors and how they specifically relate to the crew and anticipated voyage:

- Common ailments at sea (e.g., sunburn, skin infections, and seasickness)
- Common onboard traumatic injuries (Sailors frequently suffer head, rib, hand, and foot injuries, and burns.)
- Number of crew and duration of trip (This determines the quantity of medications and supplies.)
- Endemic diseases ashore in cruising areas (e.g., malaria prophylaxis)
- Preexisting health, age, and risk factors of crew (e.g., heart disease)
- Medical problems associated with specific activities in the aquatic environment (e.g., scuba diving, snorkeling, hazardous marine life, seafood poisoning)
- Medical expertise of crew (Surgical types love to stitch and start IVs; medical types favor glue and pills.)
- Access to reliable, comprehensive, and definitive medical care

The marine medical kit should be well-organized in a protective and convenient carrying pouch. Newer-generation bags with clear, protective vinyl compartments have proven superior to mesh-covered pockets. The clear compartments protect the components from dirt, moisture, and insects and prevent items from falling out when the kit is turned on its side or upside down.

For aquatic environments, the kit should be stored in a waterproof dry bag (essential for paddlers), a sturdy water-repellent bag, or a watertight hard container. A container that floats is ideal. Inside, items should be sealed in zipper-lock bags, since moisture will invariably make its way into any container.

Some medicines should be stored outside of the main kit to ensure protection from extreme temperatures. Capsules and suppositories melt when exposed to body temperature heat, 37.2°C (99°F), and many liquid medicines become useless after freezing.

When selecting a kit, think about how far you expect to be from medical care and how you will communicate with rescue or medical authorities. And remember; always know how to use what you bring in the medical kits.

CREW MEDICAL KIT

This is a conveniently accessible medical kit for treating simple and common medical problems. Keeping this kit separate ensures that supplies in the ship's primary medical kit (coastal or offshore, whichever is appropriate) remain intact, organized, and protected. Items should be grouped by medical problem, packaged in labeled zipper-lock plastic bags, and stored in a watertight container. The following is a list of suggested supplies and medications. Other brands or less expensive generic preparations can be substituted for brand-name drugs (in parentheses); make sure the crew recognizes brand substitutes—for example, APAP for Tylenol.

WARNING: A physician should be consulted before any medication is taken by an infant, child, pregnant woman, or nursing mother. Make sure the recipient is not allergic to any drugs that you plan to administer. Sharing medications with others is potentially hazardous and is not recommended. The instructions on the medication package should be read carefully before administering any drug to any person.

General Crew Hygiene
  Alcohol-based hand gel (placed in galley and head)
  Wet wipes

Seasickness Medications
  Ginger capsules
  Meclizine (Bonine)
  Sudafed and NoDoz counteract the drowsiness caused by antihistamines

Anti-Inflammatory and Pain Medications
  Acetaminophen (Tylenol)
  Enteric-coated aspirin for pain relief and fever
  Ibuprofen (Advil, Motrin) (may cause sun sensitivity)
  Naproxen sodium (Aleve) *(may cause sun sensitivity)*

Sun-Protection Products
  100% aloe vera gel and topical 1% hydrocortisone cream for sunburn, abrasions, and poison oak and ivy
  Sunblock lip balm
  Tetrahydrozoline ophthalmic (Visine) eyedrops for irritated eyes
  Water-resistant sunscreen (SPF 30) that blocks UVA and UVB
  Zinc oxide for the nose

Minor Wound Care Materials
  Antibacterial skin cleanser (Hibiclens [70% isopropyl alcohol and 0.5% chlorhexidine gluconate])
  Antibiotic ointment (Bacitracin)
  Benzalkonium (BZK) chloride antiseptic wipes

First-aid cleansing pads with lidocaine (for scrubbing dirt out of abrasions)

Waterproof adhesive bandages in a variety of sizes, including finger and knuckle strips (Band-Aid, Nexcare; New-Skin Liquid Bandage)

Nonprescription Pharmaceuticals (for common minor medical problems)

Acetic acid/aluminum acetate (Domeboro Otic) for swimmer's ear

Antacids (calcium carbonate [Tums]; ranitidine [Zantac]) for indigestion (Zantac can also be used in allergic reactions and scombroid poisoning)

Carbamide peroxide (Debrox) drops for earwax removal

Cough syrup

Diphenhydramine (Benadryl) antihistamine for allergies

Docusate sodium (Colace) or psyllium (Metamucil) for constipation

Eyewash for irritated eyes and eye irrigation

Isopropyl alcohol with glycerin (Swim-EAR) for the external ear canal

Loperamide (Imodium) or bismuth subsalicylate (Pepto-Bismol) for diarrhea

Miconazole (Monistat) vaginal cream or suppositories

Oxymetazoline (Afrin) nasal spray for nasal congestion and nosebleeds

Pramoxine/phenylephrine/glycerin/petrolatum (Preparation H), Anusol HC cream (hydrocortisone acetate) or Tucks witch hazel pads for hemorrhoids

Terbinafine (Lamisil) cream or gel for fungal skin irritations in the groin and feet (jock itch, athlete's foot)

Topical emollient (Eucerin) for dry skin

Insect Repellent

DEET-containing insect repellent (Sawyer Controlled Release DEET Formula)

Rubbing Alcohol (40% to 70%) and White Vinegar (5% Acetic Acid)

For inactivating the stings of jellyfish, Portuguese man-of-wars, anemones, and other sea creatures

Personal Prescription Medications

For all crew for their existing medical problems and anticipated complications.

COASTAL OR NEAR-SHORE MEDICAL KIT

A coastal or near-shore medical kit should contain supplies that allow stabilization of a serious medical problem or injury for up to 24 hours, until shore-based professional medical assistance is obtained. Unless one is cruising in a remote area, or adverse weather conditions are prevailing, this time frame while coastal cruising is a reasonable expectation. The coastal kit must include supplies to treat common medical problems and stabilize a more severely ill crew member in the event that transfer to a hospital is delayed. Appendix C and D contain more detailed description of nonprescription and prescription medications that are discussed for the kits.

OFFSHORE MEDICAL KIT

An offshore medical kit should be stocked to permit more comprehensive and prolonged treatment for a sick or injured crew member. Extended medical care beyond a 24-hour period or definitive treatment may be required. Although medical evacuation may not be possible, utilization of professional medical consultation with a telemedicine service, or some other private arrangement for medical consultation, along with the appropriate medical supplies, can help with medical management. For this reason, whenever a boat leaves the 32- to 40-km (20- to 25-mile) range of a VHF radio, long-range communication via satellite phone or single-sideband (SSB) radio becomes an important consideration for medical care at sea.

Don't expect to treat every medical or surgical emergency, but do not omit items simply because you're going on a short coastal trip. The same medical problems may occur on a weekend cruise or month-long trip. Drugs and supplies useful for a variety of medical problems should be selected. Above all, bring what you know how to use.

All crew must bring an ample supply for the trip's duration of any medications they take on a regular basis. Be mindful of medications associated with a high incidence of sun-sensitivity reactions (see "Drugs That May Make Your Skin More Sensitive to Sunlight," page 317) and make appropriate substitutions when possible. Appendix C and D contain more detailed description of nonprescription and prescription medications that are discussed for the kits. The following supplies are appropriate for both the coastal and offshore kit, unless otherwise noted. The prescription medications listed here (and in Appendix D) have been selected because they are easy to administer, have convenient dose schedules (12–24-hour dosing means fewer pills!), and have a low incidence of sun-sensitivity reactions. Note the useful shelf life of medication.

An asterisk (*) denotes drugs or items that are optional for the coastal kit but are advised for the offshore kit.

Antibiotics

Amoxicillin clavulanate (Augmentin) for infections involving teeth, ears, sinuses, skin, wounds, and respiratory and urinary tracts

Azithromycin (Zithromax Z-Pack) for all infections in the upper and lower respiratory tract, including tonsillitis, ear infections, sinusitis, bronchitis, and pneumonia

Cephalexin (Keflex), cefadroxil (Duricef) for infections involving teeth, ears, sinuses, skin, wounds, and respiratory and urinary tracts

Ciprofloxacin (Cipro) or tobramycin (Tobrex) ophthalmic drops for both eye and external ear canal bacterial infections

*Doxycycline (Vibramycin) for tick and tropical illnesses, beware of photosensitivity

Erythromycin (Ilotycin) ophthalmic ointment for eye infections

*Fluconazole (Diflucan) for vaginal yeast infections and severe athlete's foot

*Imipenem and cilastin (Primaxin) administered intramuscularly for urgent treatment of appendicitis or bowel perforation while awaiting evacuation

Levofloxacin (Levaquin) for *Vibrio* skin infections, and infections in the bowel (including traveler's diarrhea), gallbladder, female pelvic organs, prostate, and urinary tract; excellent for skin, ear, sinus, and lung (pneumonia) infections; slight risk of photosensitivity reactions

*Metronidazole (Flagyl) added to levofloxacin (Levaquin) for severe abdominal infections (e.g., peritonitis, appendicitis, bowel infections, diverticulitis), uterine and Fallopian tube infections, and dental infections

Mupirocin (Bactroban) cream for wounds and impetigo

*Penciclovir (Denavir) cream for oral herpes, activated by sun exposure

Seasickness Medications

Ondansetron ODT (Zofran) for intractable vomiting

Promethazine (Phenergan) pills and suppositories for both seasickness and vomiting

Transdermal scopolamine (Transderm Scōp) patches or scopolamine (Scopace) pills

Pain Medications

*Hydromorphone (Dilaudid) suppository

Oxycodone and acetaminophen capsules (Percocet 5/325)

Nervous System and Behavioral Medications

*Lorazepam (Ativan) for severe anxiety, agitation, insomnia, seizures, and alcohol withdrawal; helps with pain control

*Olanzapine (Zyprexa) for transient psychosis

Cardiovascular Medications
(depending on crew age and risk factors)
Aspirin
Clopidogrel (Plavix)
Metoprolol (Toprol)
Nitroglycerin (Nitrostat) sublingual
tablets and paste

Trauma Supplies
14-gauge angiocath for emergency
thoracotomy or tracheotomy
Eye pad
Celox packet
Full-size and finger-size SAM
Splints (2 of each)
High-compression elastic wrap
(ACE) bandages (10-cm [4-inch])
Instant cold pack (if no ice or bag
of frozen veggies is available)

Surgical Supplies
Bandage scissors (blunt-tip)
Cotton-tipped sterile applicators
and tongue blades
*Disposable skin stapler (3M
Precise 15-shot)
Disposable sterile gloves
Nitrile gloves (unsterile)
No. 11 scalpel blade and handle for
drainage of an abscess
Nu Gauze iodoform packing strips
for draining wounds
Razor
*Staple remover
*Sterile paper drapes
Topical anesthetic: LET (lidocaine/
epinephrine/tetracaine) gel or
10% topical lidocaine
Tweezers and magnifier for
foreign-body removal

Wound Care Materials
8 x 8-cm (3 x 3-inch) nonadhering
wound dressing (Adaptic, Telfa)
10- to 20-cc syringe with
18-gauge plastic catheter for
high-pressure wound irrigation
10-cm (4-inch) gauze bandage roll
(Kling or Conform)
Benzoin swabs to increase
adhesiveness of tape and wound
closure strips
Hydrogel occlusive dressing
(Spenco 2nd Skin, DuoDERM)
to absorb fluids from weeping
burns and open blisters and
wounds
Iodine-petrolatum impregnated
gauze dressing (Xeroform)
Povidone-iodine solution 10%
(Betadine) solution, for wound
irrigation use 1:10 dilution with
water
Self-adherent elastic wrap
(Coban, Vetrap)
Silver sulfadiazine (Silvadene)
cream for burns
Sterile gauze dressing pads:
5 x 5-cm (2 x 2-inch),
8 x 8-cm (3 x 3-inch), and
10 x 10-cm (4 x 4-inch)
Surgical scrub brush
Transparent, semipermeable
dressing for wounds (Tegaderm,
Bioclusive); seals out water and
allows wounds to breathe
Trauma Pads:
20 x 25-cm (8 x 10-inch) and
13 x 23-cm (5 x 9-inch)
Waterproof adhesive tape
Wound closure strips (Steri-Strip)

Allergy Medications
Betamethasone valerate (Valisone) 0.1% topical cream for contact dermatitis
*Cetirizine/pseudoephedrine (Zyrtec-D) a nonsedating 24-hour antihistamine and decongestant
Epinephrine auto-injector (EpiPen, Twinject) for anaphylaxis
Prednisone (Deltasone and others) for severe envenomation and allergic reactions

Airway Supplies
Albuterol inhaler
CPR face shield (CPR Microshield, Laerdal Pocket Mask)
Oral airway kit with assorted adult and child sizes
*Stethoscope and blood pressure cuff

Dental Kit
Dental mixture (Super-Dent or Cavit) for temporary filling, loose crowns, and broken teeth
Oil of cloves (eugenol) for topical dental analgesia
*More extensive dental kit (with instructions)

Gynecological Supplies
Norgestrel/ethinyl estradiol (Ovral) for dysfunctional uterine bleeding and emergency contraception
*Urine pregnancy HCG kit

*Miscellaneous
5-mm (14- to 16- [French] Foley catheter with sterile lubricant, bag, clamp, and plug for urinary retention; also useful as improvised chest tube and posterior nasal pack
Duct tape (many uses)
Enema bag for rectal hydration
Hyper-/hypothermia thermometer
Large safety pins
Urine chemstrips

Optional Medical Supplies and Pharmaceuticals
Digital thermometer
Otoscope (especially for water sports enthusiasts)
Pseudoephedrine (Sudafed PE) and caffeine (NoDoz) counteract the drowsiness caused by antihistamines, oral rehydration packets, or sports drinks
Reusable hot water bottle
Skin superglue (Dermabond) for topical closure of easily approximated lacerations on face, trunk, and limbs
Wound-closure forceps for use with tissue adhesive

Nonprescription Pharmaceuticals for Children

Activated charcoal (Actidose) for accidental poison ingestion

Antiseptic pads with added 2.5% lidocaine (a kinder way to clean wounds, especially abrasions)

Benzocaine (Auralgan) otic solution for ear pain

Chewable tablets for allergic reactions (Benadryl)

Diaper cream (Desitin)

ENT waterproof pocket otoscope for oral, nasal, and ear exams

Oral rehydration salts for treatment of dehydration

Pediatric-strength decongestant and antipyretic

Throat spray (Chloraseptic)

Prescription Medicine for Children

Note: Antibiotics may need to be in a liquid suspension or chewable tablet for ease of administration and dosage adjustment based on child's weight.

Amoxicillin clavulanate (Augmentin) for ear, sinus, pharyngeal, respiratory, and urinary infections

Benzocaine (Americaine) (topical anesthetic for otitis)

*Cefprozil (Cefzil) for severe infections

Several items are not routinely recommended for the offshore kit for the following reasons:

1. Intravenous solutions, tubing, and IV needles for IV rehydration may be the choice of medical professionals, but for all others training and experience are necessary. The same applies to suture sets.

2. Automatic external defibrillators are lifesaving only if expert intensive care together with a full complement of drugs and equipment are immediately available in the context of advanced cardiac life support (ACLS) and hospital coronary care units. Nonfatal heart attacks can be treated with aspirin, oral and topical nitrates, beta-blockers, and antiplatelet drugs.

Drugs Past Their Expiration Date

The FDA requires that pharmaceutical manufacturers provide expiration dates on their products. A drug's shelf life and expiration date are determined through stability testing, which ensures that a drug's potency and integrity are intact over a specific period of time. The expiration date is the date that the manufacturer guarantees the full potency and safety of the drug; it does not indicate how long the drug is actually effective or safe to use. For the majority of drugs sold in the United States, the expiration date ranges from 1 to 5 years from the date of manufacture. However, many drugs have an extended shelf life if they are stored in sealed containers in dry, cool, and dark areas; heat, light, humidity, and air cause shorter shelf life. Liquids (e.g., the EpiPen) tend to be less stable. Pharmacists generally label prescriptions with a "beyond use" date, usually within a year from the date the prescription was filled (because it was repackaged). For prescription medications going into your medical kit, ask the pharmacist for the original expiration date, keep a medication inventory with this information, keep them dry in a container, and consider using them beyond the expiration date if no newer prescriptions are available.

Drugs That May Make Your Skin More Sensitive to Sunlight

A number of medications increase the skin's sensitivity to the effects of ultraviolet radiation. These effects are termed photosensitivity reactions. People vary in the way a specific drug affects their skin's response to the sun's rays. Some may show no effect, while others develop a rash (even in unexposed areas) or intense sunburn. Reactions can occur immediately after exposure or have a delayed onset. Review with your physician the risk of taking a specific medication while exposed to the sun and consider a possible substitution.

Commonly used drugs that cause photosensitivity reactions most frequently are listed here. If you must take one of these, take extra precautions to cover up with clothing and sunscreen (see "Illnesses Caused by Sun," page 230). Oral prednisone, starting with 40–60 mg daily and tapering it slowly over 7 to 10 days, can be used to treat unexpected severe reactions.

Paradoxically, you may develop a photosensitivity reaction from sunscreens and not protect your skin from solar injury. These include preparations containing any of the following: aminobenzoic acid, avobenzone, benzophenones, cinnamates, homosalate, methyl anthranilate, and PABA esters.

Antibiotics
Ciprofloxacin (Cipro)
Doxycycline
 (Vibramycin and others)
Nalidixic acid
 (NegGram and others)
Sulfonamides
 (Bactrim and others)
Tetracycline
 (Achromycin and others)

Anticancer Drugs
Methotrexate
 (Folex and others)

Antidepressants
Amitriptyline
 (Elavil and others)
Imipramine
 (Tofranil and others)
Trazodone
 (Desyrel and others)

Antihistamines
Diphenhydramine
 (Benadryl and others)

Antihypertensives
Captopril
(Capoten)
Diltiazem
(Cardizem and others)
Nifedipine
(Procardia and others)

Anti-Inflammatory Drugs
Ibuprofen
(Advil, Motrin, and others)
Indomethacin
(Indocin and others)
Naproxen sodium
(Aleve)
Piroxicam
(Feldene and others)

Antiparasitic Drugs
Chloroquine
(Aralen and others)
Quinine

Diuretics
Acetazolamide
(Diamox and others)
Chlorothiazide
(Diuril and others)
Furosemide
(Lasix and others)
Hydrochlorothiazide
(Hydrodiuril and others)
Triamterene (Dyrenium)

Hypoglycemics
Glipizide
(Glucotrol and others)
Glyburide
(DiaBeta and others)
Tolbutamide
(Orinase and others)

Miscellaneous Drugs
Alprazolam
(Xanax and others)
Amiodarone
(Cordarone)
Benzocaine
(topical first-aid creams)
Benzoyl peroxide
(OXY facewash and others)
Desoximetasone
(Topicort and others)
Isotretinoin
(Accutane)
Oral contraceptives
(miscellaneous)
Prochlorperazine
(Compazine and others)
Promethazine
(Phenergan and others)
Quinidine sulfate and
gluconatwe
Tretinoin
(Retin-A)

*Perfumes, Lotions, Cosmetics,
and Soaps, or any Preparations
Containing the Following:*
Hexachlorophene
(pHisoHex and others)
Oils of bergamot, citron,
lavender, lime, sandal-wood,
cedar, citrus rinds; 6-methyl
coumarin

WARNING: A physician should be consulted before any medication is taken by an infant, child, pregnant woman, or nursing mother. Make sure recipients are not allergic to any drugs that you plan to administer. Sharing medications with others is potentially hazardous and not recommended. The instructions on the medication package should be read carefully before administering any drug to any person.

Acetaminophen (Tylenol) Tablets

Indications: For relief of pain and fever. Acetaminophen (Tylenol) has no anti-inflammatory effect.

Dosage:

Adults: Take 2 325 mg tablets every 4 to 6 hours. Do not take more than 12 tablets in 24 hours.

Children (6 to 11 years old): 1 tablet every 4 to 6 hours. Do not take more than 5 tablets in 24 hours.

Under 6: Consult a pediatrician.

WARNING: In case of overdose, contact a physician or poison control center immediately. Do not use this drug if you have any liver disease, or if you regularly consume alcohol. Avoid if you have an allergy to this medicine.

Acetic Acid/Aluminum Acetate (Domeboro Otic)

Indications: A solution used for irrigating an inflamed ear canal.

Dosage: Irrigate canal two or three times daily.

WARNING: Do not use if you have an injury or perforation of the eardrum (ear pain and blood in the ear canal). Discontinue if pain or irritation increases.

Activated Charcoal (Actidose)

Indications: Used to absorb any ingested poison. Especially useful for cruising sailors at risk for seafood poisoning, including scombroid, ciguatera, and paralytic shellfish poisoning.

Dosage: 50 gr of a premixed suspension as instructed on the container.

Aloe Vera Gel

Indications: A topical treatment for first-degree and second-degree burns, frostbite, abrasions, and blisters.

Dosage: Apply a thin coat to the affected area two to three times a day.

WARNING: Discontinue use if redness, swelling, or pain develops at the site.

Bismuth Subsalicylate (Pepto-Bismol) Tablets

Indications: May prevent and help treat traveler's diarrhea, nausea, and upset stomach.

Dosage: 2 tablets four times a day.

WARNING: Individuals allergic to aspirin should not use this medication. Children and teenagers who have or are recovering from chicken pox or flu should not use it to treat vomiting. If vomiting occurs, consult a physician as this could be an early sign of Reye's syndrome, a rare but serious illness. As with any drug, if pregnant or nursing a baby, seek the advice of a health professional before using. Bismuth subsalicylate may cause a harmless black coating on the tongue and turn stool color to black.

Diphenhydramine (Benadryl) Tablets

Indications: An antihistamine that can temporarily relieve runny nose, sneezing, watery eyes, and itchy throat due to hay fever or other respiratory allergies and colds. Relieves itching and rash associated with allergic reactions and poison oak or poison ivy. Useful as an adjunct to epinephrine in the treatment of severe allergic shock. May also prevent and help relieve the symptoms of motion sickness and scombroid poisoning.

Dosage:
 Adults: 25–50 mg every 4 to 6 hours.
 Children: Consult a physician.

WARNING: May cause drowsiness. Individuals with asthma, glaucoma, high blood pressure, emphysema, or prostatic enlargement should not use unless directed by a physician. Not recommended for use in hot environments, when heat illness is likely, during pregnancy, or while taking other anticholinergic medications (consult a physician before use).

Ginger Capsules

Indications: Seasickness.

Dosage: 2 500 mg capsules three times daily.

WARNING: Too much ginger may cause heartburn.

Hydrocortisone Cream USP 1%

Indications: For temporary relief of minor skin irritations and allergic reactions.

Dosage:
 Adults and children 2 years of age and older: Apply to affected area not more than three to four times a day.
 Children under 2 years of age: Consult a physician.

WARNING: If condition worsens or if symptoms persist for more than 7 days, or clear up and occur again within a few days, stop use of this product and do not begin use of any other hydrocortisone product unless you have consulted a physician. Do not use for the treatment of diaper rash. In case of accidental ingestion seek professional assistance or contact a poison control center immediately. Keep this and all drugs out of the reach of children. For external use only. Avoid contact with eyes.

Ibuprofen (Advil, Motrin) Tablets

Indications: For the temporary relief of minor aches and pains associated with the common cold, headache, toothache, muscular aches, backache, and arthritis. Also effective in reducing the inflammation associated with sprains, strains, bursitis, tendonitis, minor burns, and frostbite. Reduces the pain of menstrual cramps and lowers fever.

Dosage:

Adults: 400–800 mg every 8 hours with food. Do not take on an empty stomach.

Children: Ibuprofen is available by prescription in a liquid form.

WARNING: Do not take ibuprofen if you are allergic to aspirin or any other nonsteroidal anti-inflammatory drug. It may cause upset stomach or heartburn. Do not use if you have gastritis or ulcers, are prone to bleeding, or are taking any blood-thinning medication. Not recommended for use during pregnancy. Avoid if you have kidney disease.

Isopropyl Alcohol with Glycerin (Swim-EAR)

Indications: Dries residual water in the outer ear canal after swimming.

Dosage: 4 drops in each ear after swimming.

WARNING: Do not use if you have an injury or perforation of the eardrum, ear pain, a discharge, or a rash in the ear canal.

Loperamide (Imodium) 2 mg Capsules

Indications: For controlling abdominal cramping and diarrhea associated with intestinal infections.

Dosage: 4 mg initially, followed by 2 mg after each loose bowel movement, not to exceed 14 mg in one day.

WARNING: Loperamide should not be used if there is associated fever (greater than 38°C (101°F), blood or pus in the stool, or the abdomen becomes swollen. It should not be used for more than 48 hours. Do not give this drug to children.

Meclizine (Bonine) Tablets

Indications: Motion sickness.

Dosage:

Adults: 25–50 mg 60 minutes before traveling; repeat dose every 8 hours as needed.

Children: Consult a physician.

WARNING: May cause drowsiness, dry mouth, blurred vision, difficulty urinating, fatigue, and headache.

Miconazole (Monistat) Cream and Suppositories

Indications: For treatment of fungal (Candida) vaginal infections.

Dosage: Insert 1 vaginal suppository at bedtime or apply cream twice daily as needed for up to 7 days.

WARNING: Discontinue if burning, itching, or irritation increases.

Oral Glucose Gel (Glutose Paste)
Indications: Contains concentrated sugar for treating hypoglycemia and insulin reactions in diabetics, and for hypothermia.
Dosage: Squirt some under the tongue as needed to revive the diabetic.

Oral Rehydration Salt Packets (Electrolyte Salts and Glucose)
When combined with 1 L (1 quart) of water, these packets provide an ideal solution for replacing electrolytes and fluids lost during diarrhea illness, heat exhaustion, or vomiting.

Pseudoephedrine (Sudafed PE) Tablets
Indications: A decongestant useful in treating colds, sinusitis, and middle ear infections. Helpful in counteracting the drowsiness of seasickness medications.
Dosage:
 Adults: 1 or 2 30 mg tablets every 6 hours.
 Children: Consult a physician.
WARNING: Because of the stimulant effects, people may experience tremors, anxiety, a rapid heart rate, and insomnia. Individuals with high blood pressure, heart disease, seizures, or glaucoma should consult their physician before use.

Ranitidine (Zantac) Tablets
Indications: Relieves the symptoms of heartburn and acid indigestion. Provides symptomatic relief of stomach ulcers and inflammation of the stomach or esophagus. Useful in the treatment of scombroid poisoning.
Dosage: 1 150 mg tablet twice a day.
WARNING: If abdominal pain persists, consult a physician as soon as possible.

Terbinafine (Lamisil) Cream
Indications: Fungal skin infections, including jock itch and athlete's foot.
Dosage: Apply to affected area twice daily for 1 to 2 weeks. Do not cover with occlusive dressings.
WARNING: Discontinue if burning, itching, or irritation increases.

Tolnaftate (Tinactin) Powder
Indications: Prevention and treatment of fungal skin infections, including jock itch and athlete's foot.
Dosage: Apply powder twice daily for 1 to 2 weeks.
WARNING: Discontinue if burning, itching, or irritation increases.

Note: Among the following prescription medicines, an asterisk (*) denotes drugs or items that are optional for the coastal kit but advised in the offshore kit.

WARNING: A physician should be consulted before any medication is taken by an infant, child, pregnant woman, or nursing mother. Make sure recipients are not allergic to any drugs that you plan to administer. Sharing medications with others is potentially hazardous and not recommended. The instructions on the medication package should be read carefully before administering any drug to any person. Doses listed are for adults only. If allergic to any drug, do not use it. The warnings listed in this section include the most common, but not every, potential side effect. Update and replace medications in the kit according to expiration dates.

Seasickness Medication

Scopolamine (Scopace) 0.4 mg Tablets

Indications: Prevention of motion sickness. Same medication as the patch, but easier to adjust dose and reduce side effects.

Dosage: 1 or 2 tablets every 8 hours.

WARNING: Similar to the patch.

Transdermal Scopolamine (Transderm Sc p) Patches

Indications: Prevention of motion sickness.

Dosage: Apply 1 patch behind the ear 3 hours before travel; remove after 72 hours.

WARNING: May cause drowsiness, dry mouth, blurred vision, confusion, and difficulty urinating. Withdrawal symptoms may occur after using for 3 days.

Drugs for Severe Allergic Reactions (Anaphylaxis)

*Albuterol Inhaler

Indications: A bronchodilator, used to relax and open the small airways in the lung during allergic reactions and conditions where there is difficulty breathing. Such illnesses include anaphylaxis, asthma, submersion incidents, and severe bronchitis.

Dosage: 2 puffs every 2 to 4 hours initially, then every 4 hours as needed. The mist must be deeply inhaled, not just sprayed in the back of the throat (read and follow the directions carefully).

WARNING: May cause rapid heart rate, high blood pressure, anxiety, tremors, cough, dizziness, sweating, nausea, and vomiting. Avoid use in persons with severe heart disease.

Epinephrine Auto-Injector (EpiPen and EpiPen Jr)

Epinephrine quickly constricts blood vessels and relaxes smooth muscles. It improves breathing, stimulates the heart to beat faster and harder, and relieves hives and swelling.

Indications: Emergency treatment of severe allergic reactions (anaphylaxis) to bees, wasps, hornets, yellow jackets, foods, drugs, and other allergens. May also help relieve symptoms of asthma.

Dosage:

Adults and children over 30 kg (66 pounds): Each EpiPen contains 2 mL of epinephrine 1:1000 USP in a disposable push-button, spring-activated cartridge with a concealed needle. It will deliver a single dose of 0.3 mg epinephrine intramuscularly. Swing and firmly push the orange tip against the outer thigh so that it "clicks." Hold on thigh for approximately 10 seconds to deliver the drug. As soon as you release pressure from the thigh, the protective cover will extend. The drug should be felt within 1 to 2 minutes.

Children under 30 kg (66 pounds:) The EpiPen Jr will deliver a single dose of 0.15 mg of epinephrine.

WARNING: Epinephrine should be avoided in individuals who are older than 50 years of age, or who have a known heart condition, unless the situation is life-threatening. Sometimes a single dose of epinephrine may not be enough to completely reverse the effects of an anaphylactic reaction.

A second dose (injection) may be required if severe symptoms return. For individuals who know they have severe allergic reactions, it may be wise to carry more than one auto-injector.

*Prednisone (Deltasone and Others) 10 mg Tablets

Indications: Treatment of severe allergic reactions, asthma, severe contact dermatitis (poison ivy), and severe reactions to envenomation from hazardous marine life. Also useful as a potent anti-inflammatory drug (when other nonprescription drugs fail) for acute bursitis, tendonitis, and lower back pain due to severe disc disease.

Dosage:

Adults: Start with 60 mg (as a single dose with food) for the first 2 or 3 days. Taper the dose to 40 mg for the next 2 days, and 20 mg for the last 2 days. Other schedules taper the medication more slowly and gradually reduce the daily dose depending on the person's diagnosis and response. The onset of action begins 4 to 6 hours after the first dose.

Children: The pediatric dose is 1 mg per kg (2.2 pounds) of body weight. Taper in consultation with a pediatrician.

WARNING: Side effects include depression, blurred vision, headache, mood changes, sweating, elevated blood pressure, abdominal distention, nausea, and diarrhea. Use with caution in people with glaucoma, seizures, and heart failure. This drug can be lifesaving and is best administered with medical consultation.

Antibiotics

Some of the antibiotics listed here have similar uses and overlapping spectrums of antibacterial activity. Before departing on your trip, discuss with your physician which antibiotics best suit your needs.

Amoxicillin Clavulanate (Augmentin) 500 mg or 875 mg Tablets
A broad-spectrum penicillin-type antibiotic.
Indications: Bite wounds, skin infections, pneumonia, urinary tract infections, dental infections, ear infections, bronchitis, tonsillitis, and sinusitis.
Dosage: 1 tablet every 8 hours for 7 to 10 days. High dose for severe infections. Chewable tablets available for youngsters.
WARNING: Do not use if allergic to penicillin. Stop use if rash develops. May cause diarrhea.

Azithromycin (Zithromax Z-Pak) 250 mg Capsules
A broad-spectrum, erythromycin-type antibiotic. It is more potent than erythromycin, causes fewer side effects, and has to be taken only once a day for 5 days.
Indications: Tonsillitis, ear infections, bronchitis, pneumonia, sinusitis, traveler's diarrhea, and skin infections.
Dosage: 2 capsules on the first day, followed by 1 capsule a day for 4 more days.
WARNING: Do not use if you are allergic to erythromycin. Do not use simultaneously with the antihistamines terfenadine (Seldane) or astemizole (Hismanal).

Cefuroxime (Ceftin), Cefadroxil (Duricef), or Cephalexin (Keflex) 250–500 mg Tablets
Broad-spectrum antibiotics that can be substituted for amoxicillin clavulanate (Augwmentin) in individuals allergic to penicillin.
Indications: Skin infections, bronchitis, urinary tract infections, tonsillitis, middle ear infections, some bone infections, bite wounds, dental infections, and sinusitis.
Dosage: 250–500 mg every 6 hours for cephalexin (Keflex); 500 mg every 12 hours for cefuroxime (Ceftin) or cefadroxil (Duricef), which provides a big dosing advantage.
WARNING: Avoid or use with caution in individuals with penicillin allergy, since 5 percent of people may be cross-reactive.

Ciprofloxacin (Cipro) 500 mg Tablets
An excellent antibiotic for traveler's diarrhea and dysentery.
Indications: Diarrhea, pneumonia, urinary tract infections, bone infections, and skin infections in the marine environment.
Dosage: 1 tablet twice a day for 3 days. For kidney infections, pneumonia, skin infections, and bone infections, treat for 7 to 10 days.
WARNING: Not recommended for persons under 18 years old, or pregnant or nursing women. Adverse effects, although uncommon, include nausea, vomiting, diarrhea, and abdominal

pain. Increased risk of tendonitis and tendon rupture—the medication should be stopped if tendon pain occurs. Higher incidence of sun-sensitivity reactions occur than with levofloxacin (Levaquin).

Fluconazole (Diflucan) Tablets
Indications: Vaginal yeast infections.
Dosage: A single oral dose of 150 mg.
WARNING: Should not be used by diabetics on medication or by pregnant women.

Levofloxacin (Levaquin) 500 mg Tablets
Indications: Bronchitis, pneumonia, urinary tract infections, sinusitis, skin infections (especially marine-acquired), prostatitis, anthrax, and infections in the abdomen (e.g., intestines, female organs, gallbladder).
Dosage: 500 mg every 24 hours for 7 to 14 days.
WARNING: Side effects and precautions similar to those for ciprofloxacin (Cipro), but lower incidence of sun-sensitivity reactions.

Metronidazole (Flagyl) 250 mg Tablets
Indications: Intra-abdominal infections, including peritonitis, diverticulitis, appendicitis, and dental infections.
Dosage: 2 tablets every 6 hours if the person is not vomiting.
WARNING: Do not drink alcohol while taking this medication. The interaction will cause severe abdominal pain, nausea, and vomiting. May cause unpleasant metallic taste. Do not use during pregnancy.

Mupirocin (Bactroban) Cream
Indications: Localized skin infections (impetigo, cuts).
Dosage: Cover area two to three times daily.
WARNING: Discontinue if inflammation or irritation increases.

Nitazoxanide (Alinia) 500 mg Tablets
Stock if inability to treat water.
Indications: Giardiasis and Cryptosporidiosis.
Dosage:
 Adults: 500 mg twice a day for 3 days.
 Children: 100 mg twice a day for 3 days.

Penciclovir (Denavir) Cream
Indications: Simple *herpes simplex* infections on the lips (fever blisters), often brought about by sun exposure.
Dosage: Apply every 2 hours while awake for 4 days.
WARNING: Discontinue if inflammation or irritation increases.

Silver Sulfadiazine (Silvadene) Cream
Indications: Prevention of infection in persons with second- and third-degree burns.
Dosage: Apply twice daily to a thickness of about 1.6 mm (1/w16 inch) and continue until wound heals.
WARNING: Avoid in persons allergic to sulfa drugs. Discontinue if inflammation increases or a rash develops.

*Trimethoprim/Sulfamethoxazole
(Septra DS or Bactrim DS) Tablets*

Each tablet contains 80 mg trimethoprim and 400 mg sulfamethoxazole.

Indications: Urinary tract or kidney infections, ear and sinus infections, bronchitis. Recommended for simple, uncomplicated skin infections when methicillin-resistant *Staphylococcus aureus* (MRSA) might be the source of the infection.

Dosage: 2 tablets twice a day for 5 to 7 days

Warning: Do not use in individuals allergic to sulfa drugs. Discontinue use at the first sign of skin rash or any adverse reaction. Do not use in pregnancy. Very high incidence of sun-sensitivity reactions.

Drugs for Nausea and Vomiting

Ondansetron (Zofran ODT) 4 mg Tablets

Indications: For control of severe nausea and vomiting. An alternative to promethazine (Phenergan).

Dosage: Place 4 mg tablet on tongue immediately after opening blister pack, and allow it to dissolve. Handle with dry hands. Do not cut or chew tablet.

Promethazine (Phenergan) Suppositories and Pills

Indications: For control of severe nausea, vomiting, and prevention and treatment of seasickness.

Dosage: 25 mg rectally twice a day (for vomiting) or 25 mg tablets every 8 to 12 hours as needed (for seasickness).

WARNING: *Do not use in children.* Side effects include neck spasm, difficulty in swallowing and talking, sensation that the tongue is thick, muscle stiffness, and agitation. If these symptoms occur, discontinue use of the drug and administer diphenhydramine (Benadryl) 50 mg. May produce drowsiness, dizziness, and dry mouth.

Drugs for Eye Infections

Erythromycin (Ilotycin) Ophthalmic Ointment

Indications: Conjunctivitis and infections of the eyelids.

Dosage: Pull down the lid and gently apply a ribbon of ointment between the inside of the lower lid and the eye. Reapply three to four times daily.

WARNING: Discontinue if inflammation or irritation increases.

Tobramycin (Tobrex) Ophthalmic Solution 0.3%

A topical antibiotic for the eye.

Indications: For external infections of the eye (conjunctivitis or pink eye, or corneal abrasions).

Dosage: 1 or 2 drops into the affected eye every 2 hours while awake.

WARNING: Do not use if allergy or sensitivity to this medicine is present or develops.

Drugs for Ear Infections

Polymyxin B Sulfates and Neomycin with Hydrocortisone (Cortisporin Otic Suspension)

Indications: External ear infections (swimmer's ear).

Dosage: 4 drops instilled into the affected ear four times a day.

WARNING: Discontinue using if a rash develops or the condition worsens.

Pain Medication

Acetaminophen with Hydrocodone (Vicodin) Tablets

Each tablet contains hydrocodone 5 mg and acetaminophen 500 mg.

Indications: For relief of pain. Can also be used for relief of diarrhea and suppression of coughs.

Dosage: 1 to 2 tablets every 4 to 6 hours.

WARNING: Codeine is a narcotic and may be habit-forming. Side effects include drowsiness, respiratory depression, constipation, and nausea. Do not use if allergic to either acetaminophen or codeine.

Skin Cream

Bethamethasone Valerate (Valisone) 0.1% Cream

Indications: Relief of inflammation and allergic reactions on the skin.

Dosage: Apply the cream three to four times daily.

WARNING: Discontinue if irritation increases. Avoid chronic use on the face.

WILDERNESS MEDICAL TRAINING COURSES AND CONFERENCES

Maritime Institute of Technology & Graduate Studies/
Pacific Maritime Institute
www.mitags-pmi.org

Maritime Medical Access
www.gwemed.edu/telemedicine_solutions/maritime_medical_access.aspx

Medical Officer.net
www.medicalofficer.net

SOLO Wilderness Medicine School
www.soloschools.com

Wilderness Medical Associates International
www.wildmed.com

The Wilderness Medical Institute of National Outdoor Leadership School
(NOLS)
www.nols.edu/wmi

Wilderness Medical Society
www.wms.org

Wilderness Medicine
www.wilderness-medicine.com

MEDICAL ADVICE AND ASSISTANCE

Some organizations are available to help travelers prepare medically for foreign excursions and provide assistance once they arrive.

IAMAT

The International Association for Medical Assistance to Travellers (IAMAT), established in 1960, is a voluntary organization of hospitals, health care centers, and physicians, with more than 3000 English-speaking, Western-trained doctors in more than 140 countries. All fees are standardized. Each year, the IAMAT publishes an updated directory of its member physicians, as well as information on immunization requirements, climate charts, malaria, and schistosomiasis risk information. IAMAT membership is free. Contact IAMAT at 1623 Military Road #279, Niagara Falls, NY 14304, 716-754-4883, www.iamat.org.

TELEMEDICINE

Consultation with a medical advisory service enables the mariner equipped with modern communications equipment and a comprehensive medical kit to diagnose and treat a variety of medical problems at sea. The following companies provide 24-hour access to physicians trained and experienced in the art of remote medical care and support. In addition to medical support, some services provide training, equipment, prescription medications, insurance, and coordinated medical evacuation.

Consultation is encouraged for simple and common medical problems, as well as for serious illness and traumatic injuries. The emphasis is not "for emergency use only" but rather on early intervention and initiation of appropriate medical treatment to reduce and avoid medical complications or unnecessary evacuation.

Prior to departure, subscribers must contract with the company to provide the level of service and care they require while cruising. Subscribers can contact the response centers via VHF/SSB radio, satellite telephone, fax, e-mail, or telex.

DAN America's Hotline
(for diving emergencies only):
919-684-9111
www.diversalertnetwork.org

Divers Alert Network (DAN)
24-hour hotline specifically for diving medical emergencies
6 West Colony Place
Durham, NC 27705

Maritime Medical Access
George Washington University
2150 Pennsylvania Avenue NW
Suite 2B-417
Washington, DC 20037
202-741-2919
fax: 202-741-2921
www.gwemed.edu/telemedicine
_solutions/maritime_medical
_access.aspx

MedAire Americas
1250 W. Washington Street
Suite 442
Tempe, AZ 85281
480-333-3700
fax: 480-333-3592
e-mail: info@medaire.com
www.medaire.com

Remote Medical International
4259 23rd Avenue W
Suite 100
Seattle, WA 98199
800-597-4911
www.remotemedical.com

WorldClinic, Inc.
276 Newport Road
New London, NH 03257
800-636-9186
fax: 781-998-7954
www.worldclinic.com

INTERNET RESOURCES FOR TRAVELERS

The American Society of Tropical Medicine and Hygiene (ASTMH)
www.astmh.org

Centers for Disease Control and Prevention/Travelers' Health
Home page: www.cdc.gov/travel/
Find a clinic: wwwnc.cdc.gov/travel/page/find-clinic.htm
Global health: www.cdc.gov/globalhealth

Divers Alert Network (DAN)
www.diversalertnetwork.org

International Association for Medical Assistance to Travellers (IAMAT)
www.iamat.org

International Society of Travel Medicine
www.istm.org

Medical Advisory Services for Travellers Abroad (MASTA), Australia
www.masta.edu.au

MASTA, England
www.masta-travel-health.com

Travel Health ONLINE
www.tripprep.com

U.S. Department of State
Travel warnings: travel.state.gov/travel/cis_pa_tw/tw/tw_1764.html
Consular information program: travel.state.gov/travel/travel_1744.html
Foreign embassy information and publications: www.state.gov/s/cpr/rls

Wilderness & Travel Medicine Conferences
www.wilderness-medicine.com

World Health Organization:
Home page: www.who.int
International travel and health information: www.who.int/ith

MARITIME DISTRESS SIGNALS

1. Slowly raise and lower outstretched arms.
2. Send a flashlight SOS:

   ●●● — — — ●●●

   dot, dot, dot/dash, dash, dash/dot, dot, dot
3. Burn a blanket in a bucket to create smoke and fire.
4. Drop a dye marker in the water.
5. Fly the ensign upside down, or fly an international distress flag (orange with black square and black circle).
6. Sound a foghorn or whistle: three blasts is the international distress signal.
7. Use a signal mirror (or other shiny object such as a CD, credit card, or jewelry) to attract attention from a passing airplane or a nearby rescue craft.
8. Use handheld signal flares and orange smoke signals as homing signals to pinpoint your position once you see or hear a boat or airplane, or you are certain someone onshore can see the signal. The sighting range on water is generally 5 to 8 km (3 to 5 miles).
9. Use red flares during the day or night; *orange smoke flares are for daytime use only.*
10. Fire aerial flares only after sighting or hearing a potential rescue vessel or aircraft.
11. Fire aerial flares in pairs: the first alerts a potential rescue craft in the vicinity; the second confirms the sighting and pinpoints your location.
12. Hand-launched flares are safer than pistol-launched ones.
13. Parachute flares burn brightest and longest. They need not be fired in pairs, because they have adequate burn time (25 seconds) to confirm sighting and position.
14. Avoid using strobe lights at first: they are not recognized distress signals, but they may be useful to pinpoint the location of a vessel in distress when help is on the way.
15. Exercise extreme caution when using flares; read the instructions long before an emergency so you will be able to use them effectively and safely.

THE 15 ESSENTIALS OF INTERNATIONAL TRAVEL AND CRUISING ABROAD

1. Check with your state health department or travel medicine clinic regarding immunizations and health hazards for your travel destinations.
2. Check to see if malaria pills are required and what regimen to take.
3. Carry and use insect repellents, insecticides, and mosquito netting in mosquito-infested areas.
4. Disinfect all drinking water that is not carbonated, bottled, or boiled.
5. Avoid raw foods, salads, unpeeled fruits, and ice cubes in your drinks. Avoid food sold by street vendors. Know which restaurants are safe.
6. Do not swim or bathe in freshwater streams, rivers, or lakes in areas where schistosomiasis is endemic (see "Schistosomiasis," page 291).
7. Avoid riding motorcycles and traveling in overcrowded public vehicles. Motor vehicle accidents are a leading cause of death and injury among travelers.
8. Keep important documents and money on your person and in front of you, where you can see them. Watch out for pickpockets.
9. Do not leave your luggage unattended. Secure and close your boat when ashore.
10. File a cruising itinerary with friends and keep them updated.
11. In areas known for piracy, cruise with other boats and maintain a regular radio schedule with boats in the area. Know the potential dangers in ports and harbors.
12. Consider the risks when going ashore in areas of political unrest.
13. Register a 406-MHz emergency position-indicating radio beacons (EPIRB) with NOAA.
14. Carry a well-stocked first-aid kit and extra personal medications.
15. When traveling in remote areas, consider renting a satellite phone with worldwide coverage.

24-Hour Regional Contacts for Emergencies

RCC	LOCATION	
Atlantic Area SAR Coordinator	Commander U.S. Coast Guard Atlantic Area Portsmouth, VA	
Pacific SAR Coordinator	Commander U.S. Coast Guard Pacific Area Alameda, CA	
RCC Alameda	Commander 11th Coast Guard District Alameda, CA	
RCC Boston	Commander 1st Coast Guard District Boston, MA	
RCC Cleveland	Commander 9th Coast Guard District Cleveland, OH	
RCC Honolulu (operated as JRCC with DOD)	Commander 14th Coast Guard District Honolulu, HI	
RCC Juneau	Commander 17th Coast Guard District Juneau, AK	
RCC Miami	Commander 7th Coast Guard District Miami, FL	
RCC New Orleans	Commander 8th Coast Guard District New Orleans, LA	
RCC Norfolk	Commander 5th Coast Guard District Portsmouth, VA	
RSC San Juan (subcenter of RCC Miami)	Commander Sector San Juan San Juan, PR	
RCC Seattle	Commander 13th Coast Guard District Seattle, WA	
Sector Guam (coordinates SAR under RCC Honolulu)	Commander Sector Guam	

AREA OF SAR COORDINATION RESPONSIBILITY	PHONE NUMBER
Overall responsibility for areas covered by RCC Boston, RCC Norfolk, RCC Miami, RCC San Juan, RCC New Orleans, and RCC Cleveland, plus a portion of the North Atlantic Ocean out to 40 degrees west longitude	757-398-6700
Overall responsibility for areas covered by RCC Alameda, RCC Seattle, RCC Honolulu, and RCC Juneau	510-437-3700
California and eastern Pacific Ocean waters assigned by international convention off the coast of Mexico	510-437-3700
New England down to and including a portion of northern New Jersey, plus U.S. waters of Lake Champlain	617-223-8555
U.S. waters of the Great Lakes, their connecting rivers and tributaries	216-902-6117
Hawaii, U.S. Pacific Islands, and waters of central Pacific Ocean assigned by international convention (extending from as far as 6 degrees south to 40 degrees north latitude, and as far as 110 degrees west to 130 degrees east longitude)	808-535-3333
Alaska, U.S. waters in north Pacific Ocean, Bering Sea, and Arctic Ocean	907-463-2000
Southeast states from the South Carolina–North Carolina border around to the eastern end of the Florida panhandle plus a large portion of the Caribbean Sea	305-415-6800
Southern states, including the Florida Panhandle to the U.S.–Mexico border in Texas, plus the inland rivers including the Mississippi, Missouri, and Ohio, and tributaries	504-589-6225
Mid-Atlantic states, including the majority of New Jersey down to the North Carolina–South Carolina border	757-398-6231
Southeast portion of the Caribbean Sea	787-289-2042
Oregon and Washington	206-220-7001
Guam and other U.S. territories and possessions in the far western Pacific Ocean	671-355-4824

INDEX

ABOUT THE AUTHORS

Eric A. Weiss, MD, FACEP, is associate professor of emergency medicine at Stanford University School of Medicine and medical director of the Office of Emergency Management for Stanford Hospital and Lucile Packard Children's Hospital. He is director of the The Stanford University Fellowship in Wilderness Medicine. Dr. Weiss is a former board member of the Wilderness Medical Society, chairman of the Wilderness Medical Section of the American College of Emergency Physicians, medical director of San Mateo County Emergency Medical Services Agency, and former medical editor for *Backpacker Magazine*.

Dr. Weiss is a medical advisor and has been an expedition physician for the National Geographic Society and a medical officer for the Himalayan Rescue Association of Nepal. He has lectured on wilderness and travel medicine to thousands of health care professionals throughout the world and is widely considered the nation's foremost authority on wilderness medicine.

Michael E. Jacobs, MD, FAWM, is founder and program director of MedSail: Medicine for Mariners and Safety at Sea educational conferences; a U.S. Coast Guard licensed captain; coauthor of *A Comprehensive Guide to Marine Medicine;* coauthor of the chapter "Survival at Sea" in P. S. Auerbach's textbook *Wilderness Medicine* (4th through 6th editions); a speaker at US Sailing Safety at Sea seminars and Wilderness Medical Society (WMS) conferences; author of the "Marine Medicine" educational slide program for the Wilderness Medical Society; medical director, Vineyard Medical Services, Martha's Vineyard, MA; marine consultant to Adventure Medical Kits; a coastal and offshore racing and cruising sailor; and a white-water kayaker.

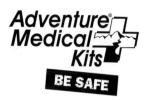

Based in Oakland, California, Adventure Medical Kits (AMK) is one of the largest suppliers of first-aid and survival kits in the world, and is dedicated to delivering the most innovative products which will keep you safe in the outdoors. The AMK team's love of the outdoors is matched only by their drive to create products that allow you to stay healthy on land, water, and air. They rely on the expertise of world authorities in wilderness medicine and survival techniques to develop and refine their products year after year. From comprehensive medical kits for wilderness, marine, and travel adventures, to survival, insect protection, hygiene, foot care, and QuikClot products—AMK keeps you safe and ready for any outdoor adventure.

Visit www.adventuremedicalkits.com for more information and products.

THE MOUNTAINEERS, founded in 1906, is a nonprofit outdoor activity and conservation organization whose mission is "to explore, study, preserve, and enjoy the natural beauty of the outdoors…" Based in Seattle, Washington, it is now one of the largest such organizations in the United States, with seven branches throughout Washington State.

The Mountaineers sponsors both classes and year-round outdoor activities in the Pacific Northwest, which include hiking, mountain climbing, ski-touring, snowshoeing, bicycling, camping, canoeing and kayaking, nature study, sailing, and adventure travel. The Mountaineers' conservation division supports environmental causes through educational activities, sponsoring legislation, and presenting informational programs.

All activities are led by skilled, experienced volunteers, who are dedicated to promoting safe and responsible enjoyment and preservation of the outdoors.

If you would like to participate in these organized outdoor activities or programs, consider a membership in The Mountaineers. For information and an application, write or call The Mountaineers Program Center, 7700 Sand Point Way NE, Seattle, WA 98115-3996; phone 206-521-6001; visit www.mountaineers.org; or email info@mountaineers.org.

The Mountaineers Books, an active, nonprofit publishing program of The Mountaineers, produces guidebooks, instructional texts, historical works, natural history guides, and works on environmental conservation. All books produced by The Mountaineers Books fulfill the mission of The Mountaineers. Visit www.mountaineersbooks.org to find details about all our titles and the latest author events, as well as videos, web clips, links, and more!

The Mountaineers Books
1001 SW Klickitat Way, Suite 201
Seattle, WA 98134
800-553-4453
mbooks@mountaineersbooks.org

The Mountaineers Books is proud to be a corporate sponsor of the Leave No Trace Center for Outdoor Ethics, whose mission is to promote and inspire responsible outdoor recreation through education, research, and partnerships. The Leave No Trace program is focused specifically on human-powered (nonmotorized) recreation.

Leave No Trace strives to educate visitors about the nature of their recreational impacts and offers techniques to prevent and minimize such impacts. Leave No Trace is best understood as an educational and ethical program, not as a set of rules and regulations.

For more information, visit www.lnt.org, or call 800-332-4100.